NATURAL
SKIN CARE

NATURAL SKIN CARE

Cherie de Haas

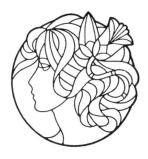

AVERY PUBLISHING GROUP INC.
Garden City Park, New York

ISBN 0-89529-400-1

616.5

Series editor: Nevill Drury
Editor: Penny Walker
Design: Craig Peterson

CONTENTS

I dedicate this book to

my mother and father –

two beautiful people.

INTRODUCTION

Health is your most valued and priceless possession. For continuing good health is your most immediate need. When sickness comes, it is your inalienable right to have a method at your command to correct and prevent problems before they occur.

The concept of this book is to give young and old, men and women, an insight into caring for themselves, to allow you, the reader, to recognise symptoms that may occur as warning signals, and know how to meet these challenges on a daily basis.

To do this, we need to understand how personal hygiene, cleanliness, a well-balanced diet and regular exercise all contribute to our general well-being.

The mind itself is one of the most vital factors in maintaining 'good health', and plays an important part in healing. With this understanding – realising that we can do a lot to improve our own lives – we can obtain not only total skin care but total 'being'. It is not difficult or costly to obtain, but the results, both internally and externally, speak for themselves.

As a child of about five years, whenever my mother was cross with me I would go into our backyard, find a rusty old tin can and mix up what my mother would tell me was a 'poisonous'. Into the rusty can went rose petals and leaves, twigs and the odd oleander leaf. I then proceeded to tell my mother to drink it all up. My mother would do what most mothers would, and played along with it. Mixing lotions and potions together was always an enjoyment for me, just as cooking is for others.

Early medicine required a knowledge of herbal medicine and of the universe. Somehow, all of this has been lost in our struggle to develop more drugs and chemicals.

By making your own cosmetics you are not using harmful chemicals. It is cheap and, with a little confidence, very simple to do.

One of the nicest aspects of making your own cosmetics is to bottle some to give away as gifts, or share with a friend.

I really don't believe that any book contains only one person's ideas; the information in this book comes from many sources. I have been very fortunate in knowing so many people who have generously provided assistance and thus made this book possible.

Francis and Reverend Frank Bennett gave me the beauty of the rose. No one grows roses like Francis. Margaret Campbell showed me so much 'beauty from within'. Roma Cornelius never 'gave up' and continued to grow younger every day, as did Ernest Clarke and Dan

O'Brien. The Clements and Barber families gave me confidence to use new remedies and watch them work. They were living proof of the wonders of nature and its healing properties. Pat Campbell gave me time and support, as did my friend and editor, Nevill Drury. I thank you all.

A special mention should be made of my beautician and friend, Fiona Bart, who assisted greatly in compiling the book, as did my sister, Chris White, a genuine life-saver. I would also like to thank all my patients who gave me endless support and in particular, my family – Michael, Monique and René – who had to put up with my absence and many frustrations as the deadline drew closer.

The oils and essential ingredients mentioned in this book are readily available in this country.

None of the preparations are difficult, but patience is necessary, as is a sense of adventure. Trying out your own preparations can be fun. This book makes no claims to miracle cures, but their effectiveness is indicated by the fact that most of the formulas have been around since Egyptian times and are still in use today.

The message that the book constantly repeats is 'prevention is better than cure'. If a person produces a cause then symptoms will result. If the cause is continued, the symptoms will persist.

Start feeling good about yourself and that will show very quickly in your appearance. Remember that 'true' beauty comes from within.

Stress is a factor in the lives of most of us, affecting the way we feel, and hence reflecting on our external appearance. I feel that Edgar Cayce sums it up with these words:

Beauty comes from within rather than as an external condition – for the external fades, but the beauty of life, of individuality shining through that personality of self, gives the beauty that fades not. As to the physical appearance and the outward show of face and figure, it is necessary that these be modelled after that of the self's ideal, that these may manifest, that the body would radiate through its inner being.

Home remedies from ancient and modern times, that are not only fun to make but work effectively, cost very little, bringing them within everyone's reach.

Many alternative practices, including reflexology, acupressure, imagery conditioning and nutrition, can improve the quality of your life in a lasting way, and the results will show outwardly.

Also of importance is the fact that we are what we eat! I'm sure that at some stage of our lives we have all heard that statement and it is indeed true that our diet plays a vital role in maintaining the good health most of us were born with. If we treat our bodies like priceless machines, they perform to their capacity. If we neglect them they become sluggish and run down. But I believe it goes a step further in that we are also a product of how we see ourselves. If we see ourselves as fat, ugly or sad, eventually that is what we become, and all these feelings show in our faces, in the way we stand and in our attitude! If we have been conditioned to believe we are bad and have our heads filled up with guilts, fears and phobias, then this will reflect outwardly. If we think positively and see ourselves as such, then the transformation begins. If we combine a good diet with a positive approach, then the results will be obvious each and every time.

So how, in this stress-orientated world do we have both? The best way to start is to understand ourselves, our bodies, our skin and how each functions together, not as separate entities.

If we are to live on a diet consisting of fatty foods, fast foods and poor nutrients, naturally it will reflect on our external appearance, like standard petrol in a car that requires super-grade petrol to run properly. If we are clogged up with constant social evenings and rich foods, then no matter how much good food we put in, it will not be utilised properly because it cannot reach the target areas. As a result, it produces more congestion, and congestion is the fore-runner to disease of the body.

Those of us whose diets are inadequate often try to overcome the resultant feeling of tiredness by popping vitamins and minerals, and wonder why the tiredness remains. If our bodies are congested then the skin, which is the largest organ of the body, will have to cope with toxins and residue from our daily intake.

In the chapters that follow, I will give you guidance on how to cleanse and purify your systems easily without going on a starvation campaign, and with regular application it will become a part of your daily routine, the benefits showing both internally and externally, particularly in the skin!

Our mind is a combination of subconscious thoughts and conscious thoughts. The conscious mind with which you are absorbing now is critical and analytical. As you are reading your mind will understand or question things. Your subconscious mind stores up all that it is in contact with, and is not critical or analytical; it just absorbs. Perhaps this is why sometimes things may really annoy us and we don't fully understand why. All our conditioning and preconceived ideas are stored in these memory banks.

I remember a patient who had a terrible skin disorder and, after a period of time, found out that since she was a small child her mother had convinced her that it was 'in the family' and there was no cure. Once she recognised this was not true (conditioning had led her to believe this was so), the condition cleared up in three weeks!

In my practice I have often seen similar cases, and I have realised that if we can clear the mind of negative thoughts, cease to dwell on the past, and see ourselves as having beauty within, the result is generally a transformation. Try to see yourself in terms of positive attributes. If you have skin problems or are overweight, imagine they have gone. See yourself as you would like to be, and as you see yourself, so you become!

It is necessary to believe in yourself before the changes in you can begin, so that you can accept new challenges positively each day. The rules below are to assist you with the positive motivation to do what you have been putting off until tomorrow.

1. Imagine your mind is a machine that heals and repairs, rejuvenates and strengthens the whole body, not only during sleeping hours when it gives warning signals (for example, while you are asleep a sub-conscious signal may tell you that you are cold, and you may pull the blankets around without necessarily waking up).

2. Believe that you are a nice person and whatever may be worrying you will be controlled with an imaginary safety valve at the top of your head. This valve will help control those pressures by letting them go, allowing the nice image of yourself to surface.

3. Imagine that inside your body the blood consists of 'good guys' and 'bad guys' (toxins, viruses, acidity, etc.) and that constantly within ourselves the battle goes on. With the attitude that the good guys win every time, imagine that the battle is raging constantly to keep us in good health. The food we eat is the ammunition for our bodies to fight with.

4. Once you have made up your mind to do all of the above, then follow them through on a regular basis to see the results.

All of us seem to be seeking the secrets of longevity or that magic fountain of youth. In actual fact, worrying about the aging process tends to accelerate it. If the corners of your mouth are turned downwards, the eyes sad, then you are going to look years older than you should. No matter how 'old' the face is, a clean sparkling skin and happy disposition will take ten or more years off your life. Thinking young is not necessarily dressing mutton up as lamb, but caring about yourself. To understand what this means, remember the importance of a positive self-image – as you see yourself, so you become!

In order to have the mind and body working together, other factors are also important. I once attended a lecture in which a very learned man told the story that Murdo McDonald Bayne had related in his book *Journey to the Himalayas.* The story describes how a young woman had a mound of dirt blocking her view to the ocean. She knew that with faith, man could move mountains. So she went to bed with her mind set on the idea that in the morning when she awoke, the mound of dirt would be gone, as she had faith. On arising the following day she rushed to the window and there was the dirt that she 'truly believed' would be gone. As she looked at it she said 'I knew it would still be there'.

The moral of this story speaks for itself and can be applied to everything in life. We have no special rights, any one of us. We have to work for everything that is really important, but most of all we must believe, truly believe from the soul, that what we want can truly be ours. Set some goals and challenges and follow them through. Be kind and loving toward people at a time when it is difficult to do so, and turn jealousies, hatred and revenge into the opposite. In a very short time you will begin to see that very positive change within yourself. It feels great and that beauty begins to radiate outwardly.

It may seem as if we have digressed away from skin care, but if we begin to separate our mind and body working as a whole, then we will only be treating the symptoms, not the 'cause'.

Each and every day, have an affirmation to start the day. It can be whatever you wish, but say it, believe it, and it will become one with you. Positive energy will create more positiveness. Most of all, learn to like yourself a lot, because if you can't, then how on earth can anyone else?

Negative energy creates sickness and disease. It is highly contagious. Have you ever walked into a room full of tension, anger and hatred and noticed how quickly that atmosphere affects you? Some people spend a lifetime caught up in a home life with such an atmosphere. Children sometimes grow up knowing nothing more. That is why it becomes so very infectious, showing in many outward signs and symptoms. The anger and negative energy stores up inwardly as well, and quite often shows up as hypertension, ulcers, hernias, bowel problems, psoriasis and many other conditions.

As I mentioned earlier, if we want good skin we have to take a good look inside as well. Keep a positive attitude, eat healthy foods, use a good cupful of commonsense and keep working on it.

Just for a moment, imagine that your brain is the headquarters for all electrical stimuli and that every cell is a universe within itself, having a physical body, a mental body and a spiritual body. Our mind determines the electrical patterns and all sounds, smells and colours are digested by each and every cell. These cells become like a memory bank, or subconscious memory, sometimes storing negative qualities that we will not let go, thus allowing them to become a habit! If our minds constantly store these negative habits about ourselves, then that is what we become. Imagine that all these vibrations being sent from the mind are filled with love and positiveness, and this is how you will quickly become.

I have watched people who come to see me, those who feel down and out, unhappy and negative, angry and sick. Once they realise that they hold the key to getting better, all I do is show them what they are really telling me. To be aware of why and how the problem developed is their first task in tackling it. Just as there is a reason for every symptom, so there will be an answer for every cause!

If your skin care routine is faultless but your lifestyle frantic, your diet poor and your emotions turbulent, then you cannot expect to get the best from your skin.

One reason that the skin ages faster than any other organ is that its external location makes it highly vulnerable to attack by factors in the environment, especially the climate. This explains why the skin requires regular care and maintenance throughout life to maintain its appearance and functions. If you neglect any part of this care, it will eventually retaliate by aging rapidly and functioning poorly.

Aging is partly pre-determined by heredity and this element is beyond human control. However, the more serious skin problems are caused by neglect and abuse, and these are two factors over which the individual has complete control. The responsibility here falls on you, not on your genes! The rationale for preventive and corrective skin care is simply to prevent or correct, if possible, the changes that cause visible skin problems. The neglect and abuse of today may mean the aging and malfunctioning of tomorrow. Skin care today, therefore, means thinking about the future.

The following steps indicate the skin's enemies.

Preventive Skin Care

1. Avoid light damage (for example, exposure to UV rays in sunlight).
2. Avoid harsh weather extremes (for example severe heat).
3. Avoid exposure to other extremes (for example hot saunas).
4. Avoid or minimise exposure to chemical pollutants and sprays.
5. Ensure good general health (through, for example, rest, nutrition, exercise).
6. Ensure a positive and confident attitude to yourself and others.

Corrective Skin Care

This involves the repair of aging or damaged skin; in these cases, corrective action is taken after the changes appear. All of us, no matter what condition our skin is in, need corrective skin care. Perhaps we need it more today than our ancestors did, due to problems such as pollution and stress. It is never too late to begin, whether you are 14 years of age or forty.

Commonsense is the basic ingredient in all corrective skin care recipes. Rather than self-diagnosing, it is wise to consult a doctor or naturopath before you apply any remedies detailed in this book.

1 UNDERSTANDING THE SKIN

To maintain a healthy, youthful skin, regular attention and a clear understanding of the skin and its functions is necessary.

Structure and Function of the Skin

The skin is made up of three layers, each of which has a function of its own to perform:

— the epidermis;
— the dermis;
— the subcutaneous tissue or fatty layer.

The epidermis is the outer layer of skin; it consists of dead and dying cells which are continually flaking off and being replaced with new ones arising from the base of the layer. It takes approximately 28-30 days for the new cells to appear on this layer, but the process may be accelerated by certain conditions such as sunburn, windburn, harsh cleansing, skin irritations and more often by sleep neglect. All of these things will affect your moisture balance in the epidermal cells and reflect in the skin's texture. This layer can easily be regenerated by certain steps requiring understanding of your skin.

The dermis layer contains blood vessels, hair follicles, nerves, elastic fibres and two essential glands. These glands are called the sebaceous or oil glands, and the sweat glands. The oil glands secrete an oily substance called sebum. The sweat glands secrete water and salts. These together form an emulsion that protects and lubricates the epidermis, preventing undue oil and moisture loss, thus helping the acid balance (pH) of the skin. As we begin to age the elastic fibres begin to sag and become slack. This, combined with lack of oil and moisture, produces wrinkling, or to be more tactful, 'expression lines'. If the dermis is starved of nutrients and bad circulation, poisons and toxins may develop and the oil gland may begin to produce excess oil, skin eruptions will appear and will greatly affect the epidermal layer. The state of the dermis is responsible for tone and resiliency of the skin as it determines skin contour.

The third layer is the subcutaneous tissue, the innermost layer, and it gives firmness to the skin. Often if we lose weight suddenly, the firmness results in sagging tissue making the person appear very drawn and haggard. Facial exercises (explained in later chapters) will assist in toning up facial muscle. This fatty or subcutaneous tissue acts as a shock absorber, cushions against blows or knocks and serves as an insulator against loss of body heat.

So the skin has many functions. These are only a few of the functions it performs. As the largest organ of the body it has a momentous job, and deserves all the help it can get.

The skin reflects our inner and general health, provides a waterproof barrier and excretes water salts, is a heat regulator and is a physical barrier against damage to the inner organs – so don't we really owe it and ourselves some maintenance?

Skin Types

Do you really know what your skin type is? There are five skin categories:

— normal skin;
— dry skin;
— oily skin;
— combination skin;
— sensitive skin.

Normal skin is the type we all would love to own – a very rare treasure, as it appears smooth, supple and soft with very clear pores free of debris, finely textured and resilient.

For people whose skin has these qualities proper maintenance is just as important as for other skin types, in order to prevent deterioration and to make allowances for our harsh climate and environmental pollutants.

Most people fall into dry or combination skin categories. Dry skin feels very thin and delicate, showing very few pores in it at all. It feels parched and stretched tightly across the bones. Dry skin often shows myriads of tiny lines, especially around the eyes. These tiny lines will later turn into fully blown wrinkles if neglected. Flaky patches may appear on dry skin and therefore should never be clogged with soap or anything containing alcohol, as this will affect the pH balance or acid mantle.

Oily skin often shines with grease and looks thick and coarse, the pores appear enlarged and blackheads are prominent. This skin type often looks toneless and muddy but these problems can be overcome with understanding. Although oily skin is some peoples' nightmare it does have advantages as well. It is the slower skin type to age and wrinkles seem much less obvious!

Combination skin is usually a mixture of two skin types. The centre patch is often inclined to be oily with dry surrounds. This skin type ideally needs two skin programmes – one for each area – with highly successful results.

Fine skin, or sensitive skin, is normally very finely textured, prone to reddish veins and patches, and requires a light consistency cleaner, moisturising and a soothing toner.

Essential Steps in Skin Care

No matter what your skin type, the following steps to total skin care improvement are essential for both men and women:

— effective cleansing;
— toning;
— exfoliation;
— moisturising/protecting;
— firmness/testurising;
— nourishing/conditioning.

If the above steps are followed, the evidence will be apparent in no time at all.

Perseverance and a positive attitude are essential in meeting the many challenges we encounter in life. Not all of our endeavours succeed, the ones you really believe in are always worth the effort you put into them. Don't you feel you are worth that effort?

Facial Exercises

Facial exercises are an important part of toning up skin muscles. The skin is generally the first part of your body to show signs of age. Crow's feet, laughter lines and frown lines are all 'character' lines, but unfortunately, over a period of time, these lines become a part of your facial structure. As we begin to mature, these lines seem to become indelibly stamped into our faces. So how do we lessen those lines and prevent the skin from aging?

Not only by skin care and what we eat, but also by facial exercises and acupressure. Certain points on the face, when stimulated will help regenerate and rejuvenate the skin tone and appearance.

Firstly, learn how to relax your facial muscles when you are talking, thinking or feeling tense. By training yourself to be relaxed, this in time will come without any pre-thought.

Just for a moment, fill your cheeks with air and remain still for 20 seconds, letting the air go with a 'whoosh'. After doing this three or four times, you may begin to feel a strain on the cheek muscles. This exercise is excellent to help diminish 'laugh wrinkles', wrinkles and crow's feet. Within a few weeks you will literally 'iron out' wrinkles.

Here are some additional exercises to help tone up your skin:

1. Put your head back as far as you can, smile, then purse your lips. Repeat several times. (This also assists in toning the thyroid gland.)
2. Fix your eyes on an imaginary spot on the ceiling whilst lying in a comfortable position, legs slightly apart, palms upwards. Stare at that 'spot' for as long as you can (6 to 10 seconds is normally long enough), then move eyes only from left to right. This exercise will help the muscles around the eyes.
3. Open your mouth as wide as possible and poke out your tongue. Do this exercise at least ten times and you will feel the muscles working.
4. With clean hands apply pressure to the area between the eyes for 15 seconds, then release.
5. Apply light pressure with left and right index fingers horizontally towards the temples. This helps to relax tension in the forehead and sinus regions. Sinus headaches can be relieved greatly by this method.
6. Push the chin outwards, so that neck and jaw muscles respond and strengthen.

Exercises should be done only for a few minutes each day. Over-exerting will strain and fatigue muscles, so gradually working up to 5 minutes will be more successful.

Facial Massage

Massage and stimulation of the skin assist its functioning capacity. If we are in good health, the skin has the ability to regenerate, cope with invading bacteria, injury, sun, wind and the effects of pollution. If facial massage is repeated weekly the correct oil and fluid balance will be maintained. People who suffer nervous tension and depression will also benefit greatly from facial massage. There are four types of movements associated with facial massage.

Effleurage movements are very gentle on the face, relaxing and allow lymphatic activity and vascular improvement. Using the palms, gently massage, increasing pressure with each treatment.

Petrissage movements are generally only performed when the facial muscles are relaxed. This involves friction, rolling, knuckling, lifting and kneading. The pressure is increased gently and is naturally more effective on mature or loose skin. On a younger skin it works on the oily surface cells, increasing lymphatic and vascular flow and thereby improving the skin's defence against bacteria. The superficial and deeper tissues are stimulated, assisting in the removal of dead tissue and waste products. This method helps to keep the skin clear and refreshed. A great rejuvenating effect is accomplished with this movement and it combines well with effleurage.

Tapotement movements are light and brisk strokes. This helps stimulate the reflex nervous response. As the name indicates, it is like a tapping movement and a very quick vascular reaction is achieved. It has a tightening and toning effect on the skin and it stimulates. Do not overdo this movement as it can produce redness and irritation due to constriction of vessels, created by the interchange of blood.

Vibrations are produced by using the arm in such a way as to promote a rapid contraction and relaxation effect. This in turn allows the palm of the hand, fingers or thumbs to produce a relaxed and stimulating result. This is ideal for fine, sensitive skin and leaves no irritation or damage to the capillaries.

The skin should always be thoroughly cleansed prior to any of the massage movements. If the skin is dry, prematurely aging, fine-lined or mature, after cleansing use some almond oil or apricot oil over the face, and a hot towel to open pores and increase skin surface temperature. Then massage and distribute oil over the face. Wipe off excess oil and tone skin with a little lavender or rose water. As respiration is increased slightly, the oil will continue to surface. Spray a natural mineral water or chamomile water over the face as a moisturiser to prevent further dehydration.

The effects of this treatment will be obvious the following day. It is also a great way to slow down the aging process. If the skin has a 'lifeless' look about it, try dry brushing in a circular movement, or if you are lucky enough to have a battery or electrically operated facial brush, begin at the neck and work over the glands, around the sinus region, cheeks and forehead. Prior to dry brushing and after cleaning thoroughly, steam the face with a combination of lavender flowers and chamomile flowers. If your skin is ultra-sensitive, loose from loss of elasticity, or suffering from red or dilated capillaries, dry brushing should be avoided, however.

2 HOME REMEDIES

As I glance around my garden and see the aloe vera plant, the cumquat tree full of fruit, chamomile and pennyroyal, it makes me strongly aware that nature offers us an abundance of plants with healing properties. Making your own cosmetics is fun, they cost very little and they work effectively. If you have some fennel, lemon grass or lavender (used as a purifier in early times) growing in your garden, pick some, crush or bruise it and pour over some boiling water. Place your head in a steam tent (towel over head) and allow the steam to penetrate the skin, opening up clogged pores. If your skin has blackheads this action will help loosen and eliminate them.

Aloe vera has become popular over the last few years, but has been around and used internally and externally since Cleopatra's time. Aloe vera is reported to have not only healing properties, but also cleansing and rejuvenating qualities. I often squeeze a little aloe vera juice into some apricot kernel oil and massage it into my face and neck in upward strokes, then place a hot towel over my face and neck. This is a wonderful moisturiser for dry skin or skin 'over thirty'.

Nasturtiums have long been used in fresh salads or sandwiches, but it is also a wonderful plant for treating problem skin, as it contains a natural antibiotic, sulphur and vitamins. It makes a fine skin cleanser, both internally and externally.

Take 10 or 15 nasturtium leaves, chop and place in a glass bowl or saucepan. Pour 1 cup of boiling water over the chopped leaves. Steep mixture for 20 minutes. Strain off leaves and either mix a little into your favourite cream or bottle and cork it. Dab onto troubled spots over a 48-hour period. The mixture should be refrigerated or kept away from bright, direct sunlight.

Marigolds are also plants which have survived the test of time in cosmetics. In addition, the flowers can be used as a poultice, for they are also medicinal when used internally and externally. Steep marigold flowers in boiling water for a cleansing cup of tea, or strain the flowers and add liquid to your favourite cream to help skin conditions such as eczema, chapped skin and thread veins. Marigold will assist greatly with scarring and aid in the healing process. Alternatively, pick some marigolds and place them in a sealed jar in the sun. When a yellow substance forms in the jar mix it with some sesame or apricot oil.

Did you know that tea tree oil dabbed on acne spots or infected skin will clear it, generally very quickly? Tea tree has an anti-fungal property, is one of the most commonly used plants in Aboriginal medicine, and is readily available in Australia and internationally.

Those blind pimples that can be very sore until they reach a head can be drawn out by applying a compress of Epsom salts or comfrey leaves. The comfrey leaves have the ability to assist the drawing while healing at the same time.

A wonderful astringent can be made from ivy. Ivy grows in such abundance, yet has so many wonderful properties. For a quick tone-up prior to applying make-up (and this is also an anti-wrinkle formula), pick 2 cups of ivy, pour over boiling water and leave to steep for 2 hours, then bottle and refrigerate.

Add 5 drops of aloe vera juice to 5 ml of ivy water and apply to face and neck. Allow to dry for a few minutes. Apply a moisturiser if desired, but this is not absolutely necessary as the aloe vera juice is in itself a moisturiser. I find this recipe is absolutely fantastic for treating cellulite. Make a sufficient quality of the mixture to cover the parts you wish to work on. With a loofah sponge apply up the leg to help stimulate circulation. Alternatively, a poultice made from the leaves you have boiled can be applied as a face pack, or on the body parts affected by cellulite.

The ivy can also be ground, added to an emollient and applied to a massage brush or a loofah. This preparation will be of value for stretch marks and post-natal repair.

Ivy is a great external remedy but should NOT be taken internally.

The following home recipes will help to restore, regenerate and rejuvenate skin tissue for both young and old, men and women.

Some of the ingredients you will need, if they are not in your kitchen cupboard, are priced within everyone's reach. Rosewater, which is used as a base for many cosmetics, is easy to make. Collect rose petals in the morning when the sun rises. They must be red petals. Place 2 cups of the lightly bruised or crushed petals into a large glass jar. Pour 1 litre of warm water over the petals and allow to stand for 2 hours. Pour contents from one jar to another several times and when the water turns pink, place in a bottle and cork it. A few drops of rose oil will strengthen it. If you wish to keep it for several days, store it in an amber glass bottle (for example a beer bottle) and cork it. This helps to prevent sunlight destroying it. Some sugar, about ½ cup, may be added, although I prefer it without.

Cleansers

This recipe may sound a little tacky, but the results are very worth-while.

Honey Cleanser
1 tsp wheatgerm
1 tbsp pure honey
½ tsp rosewater
3 drops apricot kernel or olive oil

Mix rosewater, a few drops at a time, into honey, wheatgerm and oil. Pat honey mixture from neck upwards until you reach the eyes (avoiding this area), following between eyebrows and up and across the forehead. Leave on for 10 minutes and wash off with a warm face cloth.

The effect should be instantaneous, leaving a healthy glow. This treatment is great for removing dead cell tissue, excess oils and impurities. It also helps aging skin rejuvenate and young skin to attain pH balance and moisturise.

Honey contains nature's secrets and is used in more than just culinary delights. A teaspoon of honey and the juice of half a lemon added to 1 litre of rosewater, served with spicy foods, helps the digestive system cope with any overload. It tastes good too!

I recommend you apply the Honey Cleanser in the shower or bath. I remember honey running everywhere when I first did it! A great cleanser for young skin is as follows:

1 tbsp yellow pea flour or kaolin (obtained from chemists)
1 tsp oatmeal powder (place in a mortar or coffee grinder)
good pinch nutmeg and cinnamon
water or rosewater

Mix all the ingredients together. To 1 teaspoon of the mixture, add sufficient water or rosewater to make a paste. Scrub into skin and allow to dry for 10 minutes. Wash off with warm water. May be stored for months in an airtight container. This cleanser is ideal to apply prior to showering or bathing, washing off with ease under the shower.

The following cleanser is ideal for oily skin:

Strawberries, Peaches and Cream Cleanser
3 ripe strawberries
1 ripe peach
2 tspn rosewater or chamomile tea
Crush strawberries and peeled peach together. Strain the juice through a sieve or muslin cloth. Gradually add rosewater and cream, and mix all the ingredients together. This cleanser should be left on for several minutes. Alternatively, by adding a teaspoon of honey and relaxing for 15 minutes, it is a wonderfully soothing tonic.

Cold cream is the base cream to use if you wish to make your own cleansers, moisturisers and night creams. The formula is simple and inexpensive.

44 ml olive oil or apricot kernel oil
14 g beeswax (white)
14 ml rosewater
a few drops of your favourite essential (e.g. chamomile)
Place the olive oil and beeswax in a double saucepan until the beeswax has melted. Pour the warmed rosewater gradually into the oil and wax. Remove from stove and stir until it cools.

For my daughter's sensitive skin, I add 5 ml of zinc cream for a soothing, healing cream. This cream is ideal for applying to skin irritations, nappy rash and sunburn. The quantity may be doubled or quadrupled, depending on your needs.

After the basic mixture has cooled, one vitamin E capsule and your favourite essential oil (4 to 6 drops is sufficient) may be added for an all-over light body moisturiser. For a good day-cream, add to 25 grams of basic cold cream mixture two vitamin E capsules and one drop of oil of myrrh. Marshmallow cream added to cold cream makes a great skin cleanser. It also has nature's own soothing properties!

Skin irritations and blemishes seem to be a major problem with today's environmental pressures and pollutions. If your skin is prone to blackheads or acne, try the following home remedies at least once weekly.

Blackhead Remover
3 tsp Epsom salts
2 drops iodine (white)
½ to 1 cup boiling water
4 face washers or Chux cloths
Press face washer with solution onto affected area. With a clean, dry Chux cloth, remove blackheads. Repeat several times. This treatment is most successful and has been used for this purpose since grand-mother's day!

If your skin is oily, and therefore prone to large open pores, try this tomato treatment:

1 large ripe tomato
1 tbsp yoghurt
Squeeze tomato pulp into yoghurt and apply to face, leaving on for 10 minutes. Wash off in warm water. This is also a wonderful tonic for the face, in addition to its benefits for the pores, as tomatoes are rich in vitamin C and potassium. If you wish to make a mask with this solution add 1 teaspoon of fuller's earth powder and ½ teaspoon brewer's yeast. Allow to dry for 20 minutes then wash off with warm water. This also helps to stimulate circulation and exfoliate dead skin cells.

The following is a wonderful recipe for any skin type:

Almond Milk
6 almonds powdered in a coffee grinder or mortar and pestle
50 ml rosewater
Mix all the ingredients together and shake vigorously. Strain through muslin. Babies' skin will enjoy this, as will the mature skin.

The following recipes will also suit any skin type.

2 tsp (10 ml) apricot oil
2 tsp (10 ml) milk of magnesia
1 tsp (5 ml) witch hazel
1 tsp (5 ml) glycerine
Stir all ingredients together until blended. Store in a glass bottle with stopper and shake well before applying to skin.

Almond and Oatmeal Cleanser

½ cup almond oil
½ cup powdered oatmeal
½ cup grated Castile soap

Mix oatmeal and Castile soap together, add almond oil and store in an airtight glass jar. When ready to use, place enough in the palm of the hand for face and neck, add 5 ml of mineral water and cleanse in an upward motion.

Almond and Apricot Cleanser

10 ml of sweet almonds
10 ml apricot kernel oil
5 ml or 1 tsp lanolin
5 ml or 1 tsp petroleum jelly

Using a double saucepan, melt lanolin and jelly together; gradually add almond and apricot oil. Remove from heat and stir until mixture cools. Store in a glass jar.

Strawberry and Oatmeal Cleanser

3 fresh strawberries
10 ml or 2 tsps lanolin
½ cup oatmeal powder

Using a double saucepan, melt lanolin and add oatmeal, stirring vigorously until smooth. Crush strawberries and strain juice into mixture, beating until combined. Allow to cool and store in an airtight glass jar and refrigerate. This mixture will last for several days.

How to Apply Cleansers

With a gentle motion, never pulling or stretching, and using clean fingertips, apply cleanser in an upward stroke and then outward.

1. Start applying cleanser to the neck and collar bone area up to the chin.
2. From the chin, apply mixture up towards the temples.
3. Apply cream with gentle downward strokes to the nose area.
4. From the centre point between the eyes, using both hands, apply cream left and right along the forehead.
5. Being very gentle around the eye region, apply cream in a circular motion.

Mask Treatments

Face masks are stimulating, cleansing, exfoliating, soothing and nourishing, and can be made from various ingredients to suit your skin type. They are economical and often achieve what other treatments may not. I love using a clay mask made from kaolin, fuller's earth, calomine and magnesium carbonate. If you have normal skin, the following will be suitable.

1 tsp kaolin
1 tsp fuller's earth
4 drops witch hazel
mineral water to make a paste
Mix all the ingredients until a smooth paste results. Apply to neck and face, leaving on for 10 minutes or until dry. Repeat weekly.

If your skin is dry, I suggest the following treatment once a month:

1 tsp kaolin
1 tsp magnesium
6 drops aloe vera juice
mineral or rose water to form a paste
Mix all the ingredients together. Spread thinly and evenly over face. Allow to dry – about 10 minutes – then rinse off.

An alternative face pack for dry skin is as follows:

1 egg yolk
½ tsp honey
4 drops almond oil
Gently warm honey and almond oil, stir into egg yolk. Apply over face and leave for 15 minutes. Rinse off with warm water.

If your skin is oily, try the following treatment once a week:

1 tsp fuller's earth
1 tsp witch hazel
Mix to a smooth paste, apply and allow to dry. Five to 10 minutes is usually sufficient.

Also for oily skin, try the following two recipes:

1 egg white
6 drops witch hazel
6 drops lemon juice
Mix the ingredients together, apply over the face avoiding eye area. Leave to dry, 15 minutes or so. Rinse off with warm water. Moisturise with a little almond milk, made with the following:
½ cup almonds powdered in a mortar
1 cup rose water
½ tsp sugar
6 drops benzoin tincture
Mix all the ingredients together well. Shake vigorously and strain through muslin. Place in an amber or opaque glass bottle.

Egg Mask
1 egg white
1 tsp oil of almonds
1 tsp sesame oil
pinch orris powder
2 tsp rosewater
Beat egg white until fluffy. Heat rosewater and add to egg whites. Then add oils and orris powder and mix until it resembles a paste. Apply in an upward motion, avoiding eyes. Relax for 10 to 15 minutes, then rinse off with warm water.

For those who have sensitive skin:

1 tsp calomine
1 tsp magnesium
chamomile water to mix to a paste
After mixing ingredients together, apply and leave for 5 to 10 minutes, less if you feel it is dry or uncomfortable. I have used this frequently on sensitive skin with very little negative reaction.

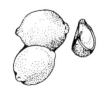

An alternative mask for sensitive skin is the following:

1 tsp honey
1 drop chamomile oil
6 drops aloe vera juice
Mix together and leave on for 15 minutes. This nourishes and prevents fine lines.

Another gentle face pack for sensitive skin is powdered oatmeal mixed with sufficient water to form a thin paste. It has soothing and healing quantities.

Anti-wrinkle Remedies

If you have fennel growing in your yard or know of some growing wild, you can use this herb, as it has been used for centuries, to help avoid wrinkles. Fennel seeds, if chewed after fatty or fried foods, will also help metabolically to avoid digestive upset and keep weight down. For this recipe, use stalk and leaves:

2 cups fennel (bruised)
1 cup boiling water
1 tsp honey
pinch of orris powder
Pour boiling water over fennel and steep for 1 hour. Add honey and orris powder whilst mixture is still hot. Allow to cool, dab onto face and leave for a few minutes before rinsing off with warm water. Apply a moisturiser.

This soothing, rejuvenating anti-wrinkle cream is simple to make:

1 egg yolk
2 ml apple cider vinegar
5 ml apricot kernel oil
½ lemon, squeezed
5 ml witch hazel
Blend all the ingredients together, apply to face, leave on for ten minutes, rinse off with warm water. This mixture will keep in the refrigerator for several days.

A little lemon juice mixed with some witch hazel and a few drops of aloe vera juice is also good for wrinkles and tightening the skin. This has shown great results from the first application. Moisturise well with your favourite moisturiser or aloe vera juice.

Toners

To help close the pores after steaming and cleansing, witch hazel (a plant of the genus *Hamamelis* that has been used for centuries) is ideal. It was used as an antiseptic and anti-inflammatory agent and I have found with some of my patients who have allergic reactions concerning the eyes, face puffiness or blotches, that often witch hazel alone will soothe and reduce the irritation. Used as an after-shave for legs or men's faces, it is not only refreshing but also closes open pores that attract dirt and pollutants, thus reducing skin problems.

This mixture will keep well in the refrigerator and applied cold has an added effect of soothing:

25 ml witch hazel
50 ml rosewater
2 tsp honey
10 ml glycerine
Mix honey and rosewater together, add witch hazel and glycerine. Shake well before use. (Lavender water also works well in this recipe, and has antiseptic qualities.)

Witch Hazel Toner
10 ml witch hazel
5 ml glycerine
3 drops friar's balsam
pinch boric acid powder
Place boric acid into witch hazel and dissolve. Add remaining ingredients and shake well until combined.

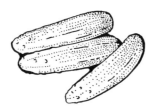

Another great toner is made from cucumber and is also very successful:

Cucumber Toner

½ cucumber

15 ml witch hazel

5 ml mineral water or lavender water

Place cucumber in blender and pulp. Add witch hazel and water, then strain through sieve or muslin. Refrigerate.

Remember that any recipes with fresh fruit or vegetable products will only keep for two to three days, even when refrigerated, so make only the quantity that you can use quickly or share it with your friends.

Once you have cleansed and toned the skin, a moisturiser is necessary for preventing dryness. A moisturiser does not penetrate and supply added moisture, rather it acts as a protective barrier against all the detrimental forces of nature; therefore it is preventive. If it gave our skin moisture, then none of us would have lines on our faces; moisturising does help to prevent them from developing too rapidly, though.

Moisturisers

The heat of summer is great but it can be very rough on our skin. The oils of sesame, avocado, apricot, lecithin and vitamin E can be added to your moisturiser or applied directly to the skin after sun, sauna or swimming. Apply these oils to the face and neck after using a steamer or hot face-washer to open pores. After you have done this, make sure you use an astringent to close and seal the moisture in.

The frequent spraying of a fine water (or mineral water) mist on the face is not only refreshing in summer, but is also beneficial in winter, as oil heaters and open fires are very drying. This will help prevent further moisture loss.

A ripe avocado mashed with a teaspoon of brewer's yeast and a vitamin E capsule makes a wonderful tonic and moisturiser for the skin.

There is no sunburn reliever like watermelon. Just liquidise enough to rub over the skin. It is cooling and soothing and helps take the sting out of the skin.

If you have overdosed in the sun, and your face and eyelids feel as if they have been starched, try mashing the pulp of a honeydew melon with a little honey (optional), and feel the relief. But next time remember to wear a protective lotion that will not allow you to burn. Far too many people are suffering the tragic effects of skin cancer.

Cucumber rings placed over the eyes will help to soothe the lids and reduce redness. I remember my mother making me take a bath in tea as a child after I had been overexposed to the sun. Try adding to chamomile some horsetail, elder flowers and lavender. Tie these in a bag and allow the bath water to bring forth their properties. The lavender will help relieve fatigue, and the elder flowers and horsetail are soothing.

After bathing, apply watermelon and cucumber to the skin, for that refreshing and cooling effect.

We may look good with a tan but it is the fastest aging factor that man has to contend with. Using a good sunscreen will help to prevent further damage. A little sun is not harmful and this level varies with different skin types, so get to know your skin!

For very dry skin, try the following recipe:

1 tsp sesame seed oil
1 tsp avocado oil
1 tsp apricot kernel oil
1 vitamin E capsule
1 vitamin A capsule
1 evening primrose oil capsule
Mix oils together and store in a 50 ml amber glass bottle. This makes a great eye oil and the throat area seems to absorb it readily once massaged into the skin. Try doing this once a week; just a few drops are sufficient for maintenance once you have established a routine.

Adding your favourite oil (for example sesame or avocado) to any good base will produce a quality moisturiser. Be careful in adding perfumes to your base if you suffer from allergies. Try a little patch test on your wrist first.

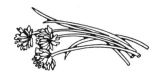

Try this easy cucumber oil for a great revitalising and protective night or day moisturiser:

1 cucumber cut into small pieces (skin left on)
4 cups water (preferably rainwater)
2 tbsp glycerine
8 drops benzoin tincture
Place cucumber into water, bring to boil and simmer for 20 minutes. Strain through muslin, allow to cool. Add remaining ingredients.

Treating Cracked and Dry Lips

If you happen to have an aloe vera plant, take off a leaf and squeeze the juice into your base cream, or apply it directly to the skin. This is a beautiful soother for cracked and dry lips. Place the leaf into some water and it will 'plump' back again.

A time-tested and proven recipe for dry lips is as follows:

1½ tbsp beeswax
1½ tsp castor oil
1 tsp apricot kernel oil
1 tsp anhydrous lanolin
2 drops peppermint oil (optional)
Using a double saucepan, melt beeswax. Remove saucepan from stove and stir in remaining ingredients. The peppermint oil gives a pleasant taste. Pour solution into jar to set. This will help to prevent chapped, cracked and peeling lips. Use a very small jar to store it and this can be carried with you for those emergencies that occur from time to time. If it melts back to a liquid form in the sun, just place in the refrigerator for an hour or so, and it will be as good as when you first made it!

Revitalisers

If you have 10 minutes to spare before applying make-up, try one of the following for a quick skin revitaliser:

Cucumber Revitaliser
Slice cucumber finely, place over eyes and whole of face and neck. Once you apply cucumber, you need complete privacy from outside

interruptions and the telephone. Wrap a towel around your head, lie down and allow the cucumber to do the conditioning. It feels great.

Pineapple Revitaliser

Before you throw away those pineapple skins, try this easy revitaliser. Pineapple contains an abundance of enzymes, vitamins and minerals and quite often the part of the fruit we throw away contains the greatest concentration of them.

Cut the pineapple skin into usable size. In a restful position, apply slices all over the face and neck. Allow 10 to 15 minutes before removing, then splash face with some mineral water and moisturise. Check on skin by doing a patch test first to avoid irritation.

Strawberry Revitaliser

Slice strawberries from top to bottom and layer over whole face. Relax for 10 to 15 minutes, then splash with mineral water or tap water and apply moisturiser.

Kiwi Fruit Exfoliant

Place Kiwi fruit skins over face and leave for a few minutes, massaging skin with fingertips. Wash off and moisturise.

Kiwi fruit acts as an exfoliant (removing dead tissue) and freshens up the face easily. Pawpaw can be utilised in much the same way, using the fruit and part of the skin.

Pawpaw, pineapple and Kiwi fruit are all perfect for making the skin feel and look 'alive'. They may be added to a portion of your favourite skin cream and left on for 15 minutes.

If your skin is sensitive, try a little patch test on your wrist first. Keep away from eye area and lips, as sometimes the fruit can sting or irritate in some sensitive or dry-skinned people. Remember to tone and moisturise skin after exfoliation.

Avocado Revitaliser

Peel and mash a small ripe avocado. Add a few drops of aloe vera juice, pack onto face and leave for 10 to 15 minutes while you relax, then rinse off and continue with your normal skin care regime.

Always avoid being too rough around the eye region, as it is very sensitive and too much poking and prodding will create stress on the muscles and capillaries.

Before bed each night, pierce a vitamin E and vitamin A capsule, mix together and gently massage around eye area. If the eyes have been irritated due to allergy or dust and wind, apply witch hazel, dabbed on with cotton wool. Then place the cucumber slice over the eyes, lie down and relax until the irritation subsides.

Eye Care

As you are probably aware the only visible living part of you is your eyes. Hair and skin are dead tissue, being constantly replaced by new tissue that pushes dead cells to the surface. With this in mind, caring for your eyes and the area around them is most important.

If we don't get adequate sleep then our eyes will become dark and puffy, the whites will begin to look like road maps and frown lines very quickly begin to emerge. So rule number one is adequate rest and sleep – this is one of the best beauty aids you can utilise. A beneficial exercise is to warm the palms of the hands with friction and place them over the eyes, repeating four or five times. This seems to soothe tired eyes, possibly by increasing circulation behind the eyes.

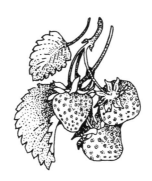

3 SKIN FOODS

If we live on a diet consisting of greasy, fattening and preservative-laden foods, then it must take its toll on our external appearance. If we live on good, healthy food, then this will show. Combine this with adequate sleep, exercise and fresh air, and a stress-free mind, and you will have a beauty package that money cannot buy.

Foods that Purify the Body

Certain foods help to cleanse and purify your body. These include salad vegetables, fruit, herbs and spices. One of the most popular as a purifier is garlic. Garlic has long been used not only to hang at your front door on a full moon, but as an antibiotic, purifier and wormer, as well as being a great culinary asset. What good cook would not have garlic in the kitchen?

People tend to worry about the smell of garlic on their breath and through the pores of their skin. Parsley, if eaten after or with garlic, will chase away the odour, but then in countries such as Russia everyone eats it, so no one smells anybody else! In fact, soldiers in the Russian army are given garlic cloves each day to keep infections and sickness away. Garlic, known scientifically as *Allium sativum,* is a member of the onion family and its qualities range from diaphoretic and diuretic to expectorant and stimulant. It has the ability to cleanse and purify the bloodstream, heal and do wonderful things for asthma and high blood pressure sufferers and create miracles for skin cleansing! So if you do not like the taste of garlic, try Kyolic or odourless garlic capsules. Garlic rubbed on acne will very quickly bring results.

The Importance of Vitamin C

Collagen is a substance that gives elasticity to the skin, cells and muscles. If our bodies are deficient in vitamin C it soon becomes apparent in skin toning, bad health, sagging loose tissue, drooping muscles and premature aging. Collagen breakdown is the first sign of a vitamin C deficiency. Vitamin C is also necessary for the utilisation of iron. Surveys recently performed in a laboratory showed that over 60 per cent of Americans were deficient in this vitamin.

Sweden has long recognised the attributes of rosehips. They contain 28 per cent more calcium than oranges, 25 per cent more iron, 25 times more vitamin A and 20 to 40 times more vitamin C.

So how much vitamin C do we need daily? Ascorbic acid comes in tablet and powder form. I prefer the powdered form, of which 3 to 6 grams daily should be ingested. I suggest starting on 2 to 3 grams, gradually increasing the amount as it does have a tendency to flush the system at first. Vitamin C is not only good for the body and its iron and collagen, but it is also a preventer of infectious disease. This has been confirmed by scientists all over the world.

Once-a-week Cleansing Diet

If an animal is not hungry at a certain time of the day it does not eat. Yet as soon as lunchtime comes, we automatically feel we have to eat. The following once-a-week cleansing diet will help to eliminate congestive foods and toxic residues from your body. In addition, try to eat only vegetables, rice and fruit the following day.

A glass of boiled warm water with a slice of lemon or grapefruit, a compote of fruit (for example, pawpaw, pear and rockmelon), and a cup of herbal tea for breakfast. Lunch could consist of boiled water with a slice of lemon, then chopped lettuce, grated carrot, onion, grated raw beetroot with a squeeze of lemon juice and one clove of garlic, two almonds, sunflower and sesame seeds, and herbal tea. Dinner could be boiled water and a slice of lemon, steamed brown rice with spring onion and garlic, then herbal tea.

Never eat fruit or vegetables which are out of season, or which are tinned, as they are laden with chemicals and preservatives.

Knowing How Much To Eat

Eat food in moderation and only when you are hungry. Try not to eat huge meals prior to going to bed, as from 2 to 3 o'clock in the afternoon our bodies begin to slow down their metabolic rate, so foods eaten later in the day tend to become congestive.

So what is the quantity to eat? This varies depending on the individual. I believe that the emphasis should be on moderation and commonsense. If your workload is strenuous, then naturally you will require more food for energy. If your lifestyle is more sedentary, then smaller amounts should be needed. Some people find it more satisfying for their needs to eat small meals regularly, rather than three main meals. If we have cravings for sweet foods, then eating small healthy meals regularly will assist in regulating the sugar levels.

If we tend to steer towards fast foods containing little in the way of nutrients, but high in fat and carbohydrate, then we will desire to eat more subconsciously looking for more sustenance. How often we see families who live on fast food tending to obesity, their skin having a blotchy grey tone. This generally happens due to lack of fibre in the diet and the congestive foods in the body, often leading to constipation, haemorrhoids and lack of energy. This can also trigger off a condition known as hypoglycaemia, a decreased sugar level in the blood.

A sensible diet would be as follows:

Sample Diet

Breakfast
A glass of boiled water; home-made muesli containing nuts and seeds and two prunes soaked overnight in a cup of boiling water, mashed and poured over muesli; one or two slices of organic rye toest with a scratch of butter or avocado butter; a cup of chamomile or herbal tea.

Lunch
Soup or fresh salad consisting of grated beetroot, grated carrot, sliced cucumber, one radish, onion and lettuce, half a tomato, seeds and nuts, cottage cheese; a dressing of apricot kernel oil, garlic and apple cider vinegar may be poured over the salad; herbal tea, water or fruit juice.

Dinner
Steamed vegetables (for example pumpkin, broccoli, carrot, potato, beans); a small portion of chicken, fish or lentils; a sauce made from tahini (ground sesame seeds), avocado and garlic mixed together is delightful poured over steaming vegetables; a cup of herbal tea.

If it is too late to eat a wholesome meal, I throw into some plain yoghurt 1 to 2 teaspoons of unfiltered honey, some chopped almonds, sunflower seeds, sesame seeds, two sun dried apricots, six sun dried raisins, six sun dried sultanas, half an apple or pear or two strawberries (if in season), and mix these ingredients together for an enjoyable snack. This also makes a great lunchtime meal if you are pressed for time.

Snacks

Nuts and sun dried fruits make an excellent in-between snack, but always remember moderation is still the key, as these snacks can be very tempting. Sunflower, sesame and pumpkin seeds are full of goodness, and usually satisfy those between-meal hunger pangs. Always grind or purée seeds as their goodness will be wasted if they are swallowed whole. Sesame seeds may also be browned with a little miso in the oven, powdered and used as a salt substitute.

Pumpkin seeds are delicious if fried in a little soya bean oil and served as a snack. These are a great medicine for the prostate gland and can be used as a wormer for children. Children generally love their taste and pumpkin seeds can be packed into the school lunch or served as an after-school snack.   Peanut butter and cottage cheese as a dip dresses up many a raw vegetable. To make a cup of peanut butter dip, take half a cup of peanut butter, half a cup of cottage cheese, mix together and use with cauliflower, carrot, celery or cabbage as a delightful summer snack. Most children will enjoy this as an after school snack. Ground sesame seeds with garlic and yoghurt makes another interesting dip.

Cleansing Juices for the Skin

Fruit and vegetable juices do wonders for a tired sluggish system, not only because of their cleansing properties, but also because certain fruits and vegetables are 'medicine' in themselves. They are easily assimilated, and work on different areas of the body. If you drink fresh juices on a regular basis, improvements in your skin will soon begin to show.

Juices may be extracted either by hand or by electrically operated machines. By using an electric blender, all you really are doing is pulping the whole of the fruit or vegetable. Grating and squeezing — for example, with carrots or onions — and filtering through muslin works but is time-consuming and not always practical. When extracting juices, remember the following points:

1. Always soak the fruit and vegetables thoroughly to remove dirt and chemicals.
2. Remove any bruised segment or spots before extracting.
3. Use the core of the fruit as well as the skin, where applicable, as this contains a good deal of nutrition.
4. When drinking juices, drink slowly and imagine each mouthful to be cleansing and regenerating.

5. Never heat juices as the vitamin content will be destroyed. Drink juices fresh; they lose a lot of their goodness if stored in the refrigerator. Buy fresh fruit and vegetables daily from a reliable source, if possible.

Nothing cleanses and regenerates the system like spinach. Spinach contains many vitamins and nutrients and chlorophyll which sweetens bad breath. If the taste of spinach juice is a little hard to handle, add a teaspoon of fresh herbs, for example, chives, parsley, basil or rosemary. Spinach juice helps to restore normal function to the intestinal tract and will help overcome constipation. Cabbage juice is another good cleanser, but add some onion and carrot juice to make it more palatable and help counteract its bitter taste. Alfalfa, carrot and cucumber juice makes a wonderful skin regenerator, as does lettuce, carrot and cucumber juice.

Parsley water (parsley steeped in boiling water as a tea) or put through the extractor, cleanses the blood and kidneys. It has remarkable properties for releasing toxins and kidney stones.

Beetroot juice makes a wonderful liver and blood cleanser. I have used this for many years with my patients. To make it you need 1 fresh beetroot, 1 clove garlic, and 1 cup grape juice. Blend all the ingredients together and drink one glass a week. Don't be alarmed if your bowels become active, as a patient of mine recently discovered after a beetroot cleanse. Make sure that the beetroot is washed well or scrubbed with a vegetable brush to avoid particles of dirt in the mixture. I blanch the beetroot in boiled water for around 20 minutes before I blend it.

Celery is high in sodium chloride and helps to pick up and tone the body quickly and effectively. Celery juice is a good diuretic and is recommended for those who suffer with fluid retention or hypertension. To 2 sticks of celery, add ½ to 1 cup water or mineral water, 1 clove garlic (optional), and 1 carrot. Blend all the ingredients together and drink 3 glasses daily. This mixture will assist in eliminating fluid that has built up and for an extra boost, add half a cucumber (rich in silicon and sulphur). Celery and cucumber juice is also beneficial for those who suffer from high blood pressure. Cucumber is excellent for promoting hair growth and healthy tissue as well.

Cabbage juice is a wonderful cleanser for the digestive tract and has a high sulphur content. Sulphur is a natural preventative for disease in the body, and also has wonderful benefits for troublesome skin. Be careful of this one if you suffer from wind, but it is well worth persevering with. If you find cabbage juice bitter, like many juices, add a carrot or two to sweeten.

For exhaustion, carrot and lettuce juice supplies iron, which is assimilated quickly by the body. Try having a cupful three times a day. Wheatgrass juice is another economical and successful therapy. (Growing your own wheatgrass is very easy to do.)

Grape juice is a wonderful cleanser and is employed in some forms of cancer therapy for its cleansing and regenerating principles. Lemon juice and orange juice are ideal starters in the morning.

As Hippocrates, the father of modern medicine said, 'Let food be your medicine and medicine be your food'.

Herbal Teas

Herbal teas are both enjoyable and therapeutic; they have been used for thousands of years as a medicine and relaxant. When you first start to make your own herbal teas, 'go slow' and watch how your body responds. Some of the following teas are best used in moderation.

Alfalfa *(Medicago sativa)* – leaves   May be drunk hot or cold, added to fruit juice or with a sprig of mint or parsley. Alfalfa helps to cleanse the system and settle the stomach acids. This tea is very rich in vitamins and minerals.

Balm *(Melissa officinalis)* – leaves   Steep the leaves for a couple of minutes; add a little honey if desired or mix with sage leaves to help clear the head prior to exams and strenuous activity. A great tea for reducing fevers and settling the nervous system. Good for the skin.

Chamomile *(Anthemis nobilis)* – flowers   Used as a tea for centuries to settle the stomach and relax the nerves, this also makes a wonderful drink for children and babies, helping to relieve colic and teething problems. The excess tea left over can be used to highlight fair hair when used as a rinse.

Dandelion *(Taraxacum officinale)* – root and leaves   A good substitute for coffee when the root is powdered and a little lactose is added. This tea assists in stimulating the liver and gall and is therefore a good remedy for arthritic sufferers. Due to its blood purifying attributes, it cleanses the skin from within and local applications aid pimples and skin disorders.

Fenugreek *(Trigonella foenumgraecum)* – seeds   A good tea to drink if you happen to suffer from high cholesterol. Fenugreek aids the metabolism and fat absorption. Used externally on acne with good results. For the onset of fever and colds, sore throats and infection, add a little honey, lemon juice and cinnamon.

Ginseng *(Panax ginseng, Panax quinquefolium)* – root   Useful for those who suffer from thyroid imbalances and as a general stimulant for faulty metabolism. Ginseng tea is good for 'picking up' sluggish systems. A little honey may be added for flavour.

Hibiscus *(Malva sylvestris)* – flowers   Hibiscus tea is a great aid in strengthening the system after an illness, during convalescence. It assists the blood with its vitamin C, iron and copper, thereby assisting the skin outwardly. Rosehips and cinnamon make it an extremely palatable tea.

Jasmine *(Jasminum officinale)* – flowers and leaves   A soothing and relaxing tea for the nervous system. Complements spicy and Eastern food and has regenerating qualities for the skin.

Lemongrass *(Cymbopogon citratus)* – leaves   Lemongrass tea has a tendency to eliminate mucus from the body, and is ideal for toning the body's tissue. Externally it may be used for skin blemishes and acne; as a skin toner it has soothing and astringent qualities.

Linden *(Tilia cordata)* – flowers   May be drunk hot or cold and makes a refreshing summer drink served with a slice of lemon. Linden tea assists the digestive system and is used extensively in Europe to settle fever and the onset of coughs and colds. This tea is similar to jasmine tea and helps to induce restful sleep.

Licorice *(Glycyrrhiza glabra)* – root and woodstock   Descriptions of the wonderful properties of licorice tea go back to the earliest times of recorded herbal medicine. Licorice helps with hormone imbalances due to its natural source of oestrogen. May be helpful if you suffer from pre-menstrual tension (PMT) or sluggish bowels, recurring coughs and colds. A tonic for the bronchial system.

Nettle *(Urtica urens, Urtica dioica)* – leaves   One tea to avoid if you suffer from high blood pressure. Ideal for low blood pressure sufferers. Gout and rheumatic sufferers benefit from this tea as the alkaloids neutralise uric acid. It may be used externally for psoriasis and itchy skin and symptoms of nettle rash.

Peppermint *(Mentha piperita)* – leaves   Great for those who suffer from sinus and headache. For morning sickness, wind and nausea, this time-tested remedy has valuable soothing qualities for the digestive system. Makes a refreshing drink either hot or cold.

Raspberry Leaf *(Rubus idaeus)* – leaves   Useful for painful periods, childbirth and lactation. This tea has a soothing effect on most female irregularities and has been known throughout the ages as a 'women's remedy'. For skin imbalances triggered by hormones (those pimples that come up right at period-time) try drinking 2 cups daily.

Red Clover *(Trifolium pratense)* – flowers   A wonderful blood clenser that increases the red cell count as it works on toning the spleen. Has been used for infertility. Add a little honey as it has rather a metallic taste. Use this tea sparingly; ½ to 1 cup daily is sufficient. A little spearmint or cinnamon may be added to enhance the flavour.

Rosehips *(Rosa canina)* – fruit   Higher in vitamin C content than oranges, rosehip tea is wonderful for preventing colds and flu. It is cleansing and stimulating for the kidneys and bloodstream, and makes a good tonic after illness. Cinnamon or cloves may be added.

Sage *(Salvia officinalis)* – leaves   An old but beneficial remedy for cleansing a cloudy head and restoring alertness at times of mental exhaustion and exams. Whereas raspberry leaf tea increases milk flow after childbirth, sage helps to dry up the supply when weaning. If you are a breast-feeding mum, it is best to avoid drinking this tea. Externally it is a great cleanser for the skin.

Spearmint *(Mentha spicata)* – leaves   One of my favourites and the first herbal tea I ever tasted. This tea is great to use as a 'mixer' for the more bland or unpleasant tasting teas. In itself it is a useful aid for the digestive system and flatulence. Combined with a little chamomile, it is safe for young babies and colic sufferers.

Valerian *(Valeriana officinalis)* – root   For those who have trouble sleeping at night, a little valerian tea (½ cup) will suffice. It has a muddy, unpleasant taste and is not liked by children. If it causes nausea, it is best to avoid it as it has strong action on the liver and increases bile. A little honey may make it more palatable.

Vitamins – When to Supplement

Do I need to take vitamins? This question is asked regularly. At times a supplement is an important part of health maintenance, but it is important to find out exactly which ones are needed. So often we read an article that says if you have a particular symptom then you need this or that vitamin. Firstly, ask yourself why is your body deficient in it anyway, and what is the cause? Have this checked up first by visiting your doctor and naturopath. Missing vitamins or minerals can often be replaced by eating the foods that contain them.

People who are taking tablets for blood pressure are often supplemented with potassium as diuretics (fluid tablets) cause, in some cases, a loss of potassium and this can bring on many symptoms. As an Indian surgeon who recently lectured on minerals said, 'If soil is severely deficient in potassium, then the plants and trees often grow mutated or develop lumps on the trunk. They rarely survive or look healthy'. So if our systems are potassium deficient, skin disorders, rashes and eczema can often result, not to mention tiredness and lethargy which can trigger off depression, and so the vicious circle continues. Always try to take potassium in its natural form, as it can be dangerous if self-administered or administered incorrectly. Some of the best sources for potassium are dried apricots, bananas, lentils, figs and spinach.

To find if you are deficient in any vitamins or minerals, hair analysis is worthy of a mention. Hair analysis, generally conducted at pathology units, is a little like comparing your hair with the leaves on a tree. If the tree is strong and healthy and living in the right conditions, the leaves will be likewise. Our hair is the first noticeable part of our physical body to suffer, as well as our skin, if conditions internally are not strong and healthy. Hair analysis will show not only what we are deficient in at the time of the analysis, but also what we are excessive in. One of my patients has cancer. Her doctor, who is treating her for such, found high levels of aluminium, lead and arsenic in her analysis. Where do these come from? The pathologist suggested that pollution, fruit and vegetable sprays and aluminium cookware all contributed greatly. So vitamin deficiencies are not always at the root of health problems.

4 FROM THE GARDEN TO THE SKIN

A comprehensive description of all the parts with therapeutic qualities could fill a library of books. In this chapter I will simply discuss some of the plants which provide benefits for the skin as well as for other facets of health. These plants are readily available and may easily be grown in your garden – fresh from the garden is of course the best way to use them.

Watercress *(Nasturtium officinale),* found in many gardens and often along creek beds, contains vitamins A and E and has an abundance of minerals. The juice of the watercress applied to the face will help to treat spots and pimples; it can be left on overnight. The seeds of the watercress contain mustard oil, so watercress has the most to offer when the plant is in flower.

I recently advised a patient, who had many acne spots on her face, to try dabbing the juice of the watercress onto her skin. Within a week the improvement was quite dramatic. I feel the sulphur, iodine, iron, vitamins and minerals that constitute watercress have been long overlooked.

Sweet violets *(Viola odorata)* are another old and proven remedy, used both internally and externally. When I was working in the far north of Queensland, where nature's resources for medicine are abundant, I came across a very sick young woman with glandular fever. The only resources at hand were the fresh, healthy sweet violets growing in her garden. After brewing up the whole of the plant and making it into a tea, small doses were administered frequently and this gradually seemed to assist her recovery, as the violet tea reduced the fever. The flowers of the violet, after being saturated with wine or water, can be applied to the skin to ease rheumatic pain, eruptions or any skin problem that seems to need a soothing and cooling effect. In cases of psoriasis and eczema the heat will be eased greatly if violet water or wine is applied. A compress to the liver in cases of glandular fever will also assist.

Lemon verbena *(Lippia citriodora)* is one of the most pleasant tasting and medicinally beneficial plants. The perfume of the lemon verbena has been incorporated into cosmetics, herbal sachets and potpourris for many years. Lemon verbena is said to aid tone to the skin as it stimulates. Internally it helps relieve wind and stomach upsets, and if you are having trouble with any of these it is certainly

worth trying a cup of lemon verbena together for a delightfully different and healthy cup of tea. This is also lovely cold in summer with a
slice of orange, lemon or lime. Remember that herbs can be used and
often the second filling of the teapot has given the herbs time to expel
their various properties and the second pouring can often be a lot
stronger. The quantity of herbs depends on how strong or mild you
prefer the tea. Generally 1 to 2 teaspoons of the dry herb per person
is sufficient. If the herb is freshly picked, at least double the quantity.

Parsley *(Petroselinum crispun)* has many, many uses in the kitchen
and in medicine. It was utilised in World War I for the soldiers who
were constantly getting dysentery and kidney infections. It has a calming action and soothing effect on the nervous system, and as a diuretic the benefits are wonderful. High-blood pressure patients should
try a daily cup of parsley tea. It also contains iron and vitamin C,
amongst its many minerals and vitamins.

I see so many people leave their parsley decorations lying on the
side of their plate. If the truth be known, they have probably thrown
away the most nutritious part of the whole meal.

As mentioned earlier, parsley makes a great garlic chaser and
commercially made garlic tablets often contain parsley. Both garlic
and parsley aid in treatment of hypertension, so try to utilise them in
your daily diet.

Parsley grown in pots in the kitchen or on the verandah not only
looks lovely but is encouragingly handy to cook with or nibble on. I
find it helpful when one suffers from nausea or morning sickness, and
the benefits go on and on. Herbalists in former times used it extensively in removing gravel from the kidneys, and old medical records
confirm that some of our former doctors of medicine used or recommended it quite frequently.

When you start experimenting with the internal use of various
herbs, be very sure you understand what they are and what they do.
Herbs react on different people in many different ways and for this
reason you could make yourself quite ill if you overdose on
too many strong herbs. Moderation in everything is absolutely
essential.

Sage *(Salvia officinalis)* has many benefits. Sage leaves rubbed onto
the gums will help with bleeding and inflammation. A wonderful
mouth freshener can be made by adding a handful of spearmint

leaves to 1 cup of sage leaves, bruising them and pouring over 2 cups of boiled water. Bottle in a sterile jar and refrigerate. Make a fresh batch every two days. Cinnamon water may be added and I find a quarter of a stick of cinnamon dissolved in approximately 1 cup of boiled water is sufficient. A gargle for sore throats and mouth ulcers can be used with the same recipe; it brings very quick relief.

Fennel *(Foeniculum vulgare).* Chewing on fennel seeds (or alternatively peppermint or spearmint leaves or wheat grass) will freshen up a stale breath. Fennel seeds will help the digestive tract as they work on the liver, spleen and gall bladder. Some of my patients chew them for indigestion or heartburn. Others swear by them for wind and keeping off those excess pounds, if chewed after meals. Fennel seeds complement fish meals and taken after fatty foods, settle the stomach.

Chamomile *(Anthemis nobilis),* mentioned earlier as a beneficial herbal tea, can be used both internally and externally. It is often recommended for stomach complaints and frequently assists little children and babies when they are teething, have stomach upsets or are irritable. Chamomile has a distinct aroma which can be likened to that of apples. The Egyptians used it constantly in medicine and today more people are becoming aware of its value. It is extremely successful for period pain and gripping pain. A cup of chamomile tea and a bath in chamomile will assist greatly with hysteria, both internal and external effects. To make a soothing lotion for inflamed, itchy or dry skin, try some chamomile lotion. Pick a cupful of flowers and leaves, crush and pour over 1 litre of boiling water, and allow to steep for 1 hour. With clean hands and cotton wool or a face washer, wash face or dab onto affected areas. The remainder may be put into your bath or used as a hair rinse to add life and lustre.

Chamomile has the ability to soothe toothache and abscesses. Make a little muslin or cloth bag and place chamomile flowers loosely into it. Soak in boiling water and then apply to the area that is inflamed. I find this remedy also assists in reducing swollen glands. I recently advised a young mother whose two-year-old son was suffering great discomfort with mumps, to apply a chamomile bag to the painful areas. Three days later she claimed it had assisted greatly and he also seemed to sleep more peacefully once it had been applied. A warm solution was given internally at the same time and this would have helped to calm the nervous system.

Couch grass *(Agropyron repens)*. Would you believe that common couch grass has many benefits for the skin? Couch grass is also one of nature's remedies for cats, dogs and horses. If they are not feeling in peak condition they are often seen eating grasses. Today peasants in some countries still gather couch grass from sandy banks and sell it as medicine! The juicy roots of the grass have a sweet pleasant taste and can be used internally and externally.

After picking around 2 cups of couch grass (the straw-coloured roots being the most beneficial part), pour 1 litre of boiling water over, steep and drink as a cleansing tea. This is also very beneficial for the liver. In addition, couch grass has been applied successfully for urinary tract infections and kidney stones. If the liver and kidneys are not functioning up to par, then the skin will suffer from the poisons and toxins left in the blood, leaving it blotchy and sallow. Couch grass can be applied to acne and inflamed skin as a lotion or as a strong infusion which can be mixed into a base cream and applied as a day cream. It has diuretic and antibiotic properties and has been used as a treatment for rheumatic pain. So, before you curse the couch grass taking over your garden, remember its great medicinal value.

For a very strong, once-daily cleanser for the blood, kidneys and liver, the following recipe will have you moving!

½ cup couch grass roots
½ cup parsley
½ cup of dandelion roots
The roots of the dandelions can be chopped and expressed by allow-ing them to stand in cold water for 2 hours and then boiling them for 10 minutes. Bruise the couch grass roots and parsley and pour 1 litre of boiled dandelion root water over them. The tea may be taken hot or cold; the couch grass seems to give it a pleasant sweet taste. (The dandelion helps to stimulate secretions in the glands and assists the pancreas and bile ducts.)

Horsetail *(Equisetum arvense)*. The dried green shoots of the horse-tail can be applied externally for wounds and sores that tend to heal slowly. Eruptions and boils respond well to a poultice made from horsetail. Squeeze juice from the freshly picked plant and apply to the affected area; a few drops will suffice. Repeat this action twice daily. This may be used to treat pimples and skin eruptions, and cracking, brittle nails benefit greatly from it as well.

Arnica (*Arnica montana*) has long been used in medicine. Most of our grandmothers had arnica on hand for bruising or skin eruptions. It was used for throat and mouth infections in the form of a gargle. Use internally only with supervision from your homeopath or herbalist, as it is toxic. It is used most safely as a compress or as a liniment for sprains, strains and rheumatism. I find the best method, after collecting the flower heads, is to dry them in a shady spot; to 1 cup of flowers, pour over ½ litre of boiling water, steep and use as a compress. For skin eruptions, mix 10 drops of arnica to 10 drops of aloe vera juice and dab on problem skin areas. Arnica used as a compress for chilblains has a remarkable affect. It will irritate if repeated too frequently, however.

Marigold (*Calendula officinalis*). How I love this beautiful plant! It has brought me many positive results through its ability to heal. The flowers and leaves are used. Mrs Grieve, in her book *A Modern Herbal,* suggests that the flower be rubbed onto the area where a wasp or bee has stung, to help to reduce pain and swelling. For wounds and skin eruptions, marigolds are in a class of their own. I have seen many cases of eczema and psoriasis respond to calendula cream and I incorporate it often into an arnica-based cold cream. Dry the flowers in a shady position, place in a mortar and pestle or a coffee grinder, and reduce to a powder. The powder can be mixed in creams or in distilled water and strained through muslin.

Horseradish (*Cochlearia armoracia*) has been used for centuries both as a culinary delight and for poultices. The root of the horseradish is the part most commonly used and this, when infused in hot milk, makes a soothing and stimulating tonic for the skin. The root contains high quantities of sulphur and this acts as a natural deterrent to skin problems. It has been used for centuries for gout, neuralgia, rheumatism, swellings and joint pains. A poultice may be used by scraping the root and applying to areas in need, then binding with a bandage; this will bring great relief. A patient recently claimed that she had 'cured' rheumatic pains in her wrist by securing freshly scraped horseradish root onto a piece of tape, and then lightly bandaging both wrists. Within a couple of days all pain had gone. Small internal doses were then taken, and she noticed her stomach and wind seemed to settle. (It is known to be a wonderful stimulant to the digestive system.)

If taken with some garlic, horseradish assists congestion in the nasal passages and breaks down catarrh. Health food shops generally stock tablets for sinus and hayfever which are a combination of horseradish and garlic.

St John's Wort *(Hypericum perforatum)*. To make a lotion for cuts and wounds, this is ideal. Pick a handful of the golden yellow flowers, bruise them and place in 50 ml of olive oil. Leave to steep for a couple of days and apply to the skin. A few drops applied to dry skin, chapped hands and cracked skin works wonders. This can be safely applied to eczema and psoriasis. It yields the soothing and healing quality.

Collection of Herbs and Flowers

The best time to collect herbs and flowers for drying is just after the sun has been up long enough to have dried the dew from the grasses and plants. Choose a sunny day when the weather has been gentle on the flowers and they are not already bruised and torn. To prevent dampness and mould forming, remove all leaves and flowers from the stems and spread out on mesh or wire in a room that is airy and not damp.

If you need to hang them, separate into small bunches and hang from a beam or ceiling. Mint, parsley and lavender dry well this way. The leaves and flowers that retain much of their natural colour will yield the strongest odour generally.

Gathering your own herbs and flowers can be quite an event. If you are selecting plants from the mountains or the bush, a linen bag or a cane basket is ideal. Plastic bags sweat, and you may lose the quality of the plant before you get home. Only collect what you need, with a good pair of garden secateurs or scissors. Collecting can be half the pleasure of making your own cosmetics and skin care items, so select carefully and enjoy it. Once dried, store the plants in an airtight container.

To collect seeds, gather them when they are fully ripe, dry and store in an airtight container until required.

Bulbs should be collected after the leaves have died off the stem. Slice the bulb after removing the outer layer. It can be dried in the oven on a low heat, or placed in the oven when it is retaining heat after previous use. Dry until the bulb becomes brittle. Bark can be dried in the sunlight or gathered, tied and stored in a cane basket or hung outside in the sunlight. If the bark is rough, shave or smooth down before drying and use the inner bark.

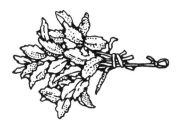

5 THE MAGIC OF OILS

Oils derived from plants have been used since ancient times, not only for their exquisite fragrances, but also because of their proven effectiveness in treating a wide variety of health problems, including those concerning the skin.

Aromatherapy

Many countries are now practising the art of aromatherapy, a gentle science based on the use of essential oils derived from flowers, trees, herbs and resins. These are used to treat the skin, to stimulate or relax, and to maintain bodily resistance to disease. Essential oils are considered the 'life force', sometimes even the 'soul' of the plant, and thus transmit a living energy to a person. This is generally achieved by massaging the oils into the skin, adding them to a warm bath, inhaling them or taking them internally.

Each practitioner uses his own discretion as to which oils are suitable for a person, as it is considered that a patient's basic chemical state is determined by individual physiology and personality. By absorption through the skin or by taking internally, the oils pass through the body to various key areas. Scientific research has revealed that traces of essential oil, after being placed on a shaved part of a rat, were found in the kidneys at dissection after one hour. Qualified medical doctors are the only people allowed to practise aromatherapy in France, where it may be studied as a university course.

The ancient Egyptians, Greeks, Chinese and Indians realised the vital roles of oils as antiseptics and purifiers, and for embalming. Their secrets were closely guarded and laboratories were set up so that experiments of different kinds could be performed with barks, seeds, flowers and roots. Some plants were held sacred, for example the lotus flower was revered in India as it was supposed to have been the first living plant to appear on the earth. It was believed that as its petals unfurled the supreme God of the Intellect was revealed. Lotus oil is widely used today for its fragrance and the flower is still held in awe because of its sheer beauty.

Unlike other oils, essential oils are absorbed into the blood supply via the pores which produce sweat and sebum. Just as homeopathic remedies find their way to the part of the body in need of help, these oils go to work in the kidney region, liver or nervous system, or any other part where they are needed. As an indication of the way in which these oils pass through the body, try placing a few drops of garlic oil on the soles of the feet; within a couple of hours, it can be tasted or smelt on the breath.

Most essences are cell-regenerating and stimulating. Lavender oil in particular has a rejuvenating effect, and one only has to watch skin that has been burnt respond to lavender oil, to note its effects. Fennel oil is an anti-wrinkle oil; it contains oestrogens that suit the more mature skin. (Add a little myrrh oil to camouflage the fennel odour.) A list of various oils and their uses is included in Chapter 12.

Generally it is advisable to use 1 per cent to 5 per cent essential oils with a base such as apricot, avocado or sesame oil (or other oil which has no perfume). Camphor, pennyroyal and cedarwood oil should be avoided by pregnant women, both internally and externally, and a substitute incorporated: for example, lavender or rose. As the oils are powerful in their properties when taken internally, one or two drops is usually sufficient three times daily on a little sugar or a sugar pill. Do not take oil internally if you are on homeopathic treatment without first checking with your practitioner.

Acne

If you suffer from acne, a massage oil will benefit. This treatment should be applied daily; be persistent and the results will show.

50 ml base of apricot oil
10 drops lemon oil
10 drops cypress oil
5 drops lavender oil
Combine the oils and massage well into lymph glands (down both sides of the neck), sinus region and forehead.

Also good for acne is lavender oil, used for its antiseptic qualities, diluted in witch hazel and dabbed onto the skin.

Tea tree oil, applied directly onto acne spots, acts as an antifungal. I have seen it achieve some amazing results. Lemongrass oil can also be applied directly onto acne as a beneficial treatment.

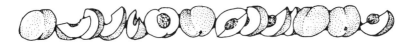

Dry Skin

Dry skin will be helped by the following mixtures:

— geranium oil: 20 drops to 50 ml apricot oil;
— sandalwood oil: 20 drops to 50 ml apricot oil;
— rose oil: 20 drops to 50 ml apricot oil;
— rose geranium oil: 20 drops to 50 ml of apricot oil;
— ylang-ylang oil: 10 drops mixed with 10 drops of lavender oil in
   50 ml apricot oil;
—· petitgrain oil: 20 drops to 50 ml apricot oil;
— rosemary oil: 20 drops to 50 ml apricot oil.

The following formula is another treat for dry skin:

50 ml sesame oil
10 drops sandalwood oil
8 drops geranium oil
5 drops lavender oil
5 drops rosewood oil
2 drops ylang-ylang oil
After cleansing the face and neck, tone the skin with your toner. Some people prefer to spray with a little mineral water before applying massage oil. Massage well into face and neck before retiring, avoiding at all times the eye area. The essential oils work best when you are in a relaxed state. Do this at least two to three times a week and your skin will show the benefits.

Oily Skin

The oils used for oily skin are generally the same as those used for acne. A hot compress applied over the face will help open pores. Always follow with a toner to close off the open pores. Witch hazel will suffice in this case or warm water and lemon juice. This is also great as an after shave bracer.

Mature Skin

For the mature lady, the following is beneficial:

30 ml sesame oil
10 ml jojoba oil
4 drops Neroli oil
2 drops frankincense oil
1 drop ylang-ylang oil
Apply this each night before retiring and the difference will be obvious within a few weeks.

The following two remedies will also improve the appearance of mature skin:

4 drops Neroli oil
10 drops lavender oil
30 drops jojoba oil
10 drops glycerine oil
60 drops castor oil
Mix all the ingredients together and apply a few drops to the face and neck. Apply a hot flannel as a compress.

1 vitamin E capsule 500 IU
1 vitamin A capsule 10 000 IU
5 ml apricot kernel oil
2 drops lavender oil
1 drop myrrh oil
10 drops glycerine oil
Stir all the ingredients together and store in a small amber bottle approximately 25 ml in size. If placed in a decorative bottle, it makes a very appealing gift.

Eye and Throat

This is a delicate oil and a wonderful skin regenerator for the eye and throat areas:

1 drop myrrh oil
1 drop frankincense oil

10 ml glycerine
10 ml castor oil
(This will feel like a very thick egg white, as it is of heavier consistency.) With clean fingertips gently stroke oil around eyes and out
towards the ears from the bridge of the nose. Massage upwards from
collar bone to chin. Repeat nightly.

The following is also excellent for the skin around the eyes and the
throat area:

3 drops Neroli oil
2 drops myrrh oil
1 drop lotus oil
30 drops jojoba oil
10 ml glycerine
50 ml apricot kernel oil
To produce a massage oil, combine all of these oils.

Psoriasis

This is a remedy for the treatment of the skin disorder known as
psoriasis:

2 drops cajuput oil
2 drops calendula oil
1 drop oregano
2 drops lavender oil
50 ml castor oil or 25 ml jojoba oil
25 ml apricot oil
Mix all the ingredients together and massage over affected area.
Alternatively, a few drops can be added to your bath.

Burns and Scalds

Lavender oil may be used to treat burns and scalds by applying
directly. Alternatively, steep some lavender flowers, soak bandages in
the solution and apply as a compress.
    The juice of the aloe vera plant can be applied directly to burns.
Comfrey leaves or elder flowers, bruised and steeped, may be applied
as a compress.

Staph Sores

Sandalwood oil in a teaspoon of buttercup juice may be applied to these sores. Alternatively, the sandalwood oil may be diluted in 50 ml olive oil, a compress soaked in the solution and applied to the sore.

Sunburn

Lavender oil, applied often, is as effective for sunburn as it is for burns and scalds. Dilute 25 drops of lavender oil in 50 ml apricot oil. Aloe vera juice may also be applied to the affected areas.

Alternatively, mix together and apply to the skin 12 drops of balm of Gilead (also known as balsam), 10 drops of elder flower oil, 15 drops of calendula oil, and 50 ml of castor oil. In biblical times balm of Gilead was used in cosmetics. The buds of the plant from which it is derived, *Commiphora opobalsamum,* may be steeped in rum and applied to heal cuts and bruises. A compress soaked in the rum and flower mixture can also be applied to psoriasis or sunburnt areas.

Itchy Skin and other Irritations

Mix together 20 drops of bay laurel oil and 50 ml castor oil. Apply directly to the irritation and it will soon bring relief. Parsley oil, rosemary or sage oil will also suffice, or a combination of all together will be beneficial. One of my own concoctions has worked successfully many times : to 50 ml castor oil add 5 drops of oil of bay, 10 drops of calendula oil, 5 drops of thuja oil and 5 drops of myrrh oil, and apply to irritated areas.

Feet

For those who would like their feet and shoes to smell fresh, even during those hot, sticky summer days, the following deodorant is recommended :

Foot Powder Deodorant
2 cups dried lavender flowers or 20 drops oil of lavender
25 g (1 oz) orris root powder
50 g (2 oz) arrowroot
Grind lavender flowers to a powder in a mortar or coffee grinder. Mix

orris root powder and arrowroot into lavender powder and add lavender oil. Sprinkle a little in shoes and rub powder over feet and between toes.

If you happen to be one of the millions of people who suffer from tinea or athlete's foot, this seems to be a 'never fail' remedy.

Athlete's Foot Lotion
1 tbsp chamomile flowers
4 drops myrrh oil
3 drops benzoin
60 drops vodka
200 ml boiling water

Myrrh and Sandalwood Oil for Feet
20 drops witch hazel
3 drops myrrh oil
3 drops sandalwood oil
2 drops benzoin
30 ml lavender oil
30 ml lavender water
Mix all the ingredients. Soak a piece of cotton in the solution and place inside shoe or stocking. This will continue acting as a deodoriser all day.

If your feet are rough, and hard skin seems to make your feet unsightly, soak feet in a shallow bath with Epsom salts. With a pumice stone or nail brush, rub gently on rough skin area, followed by a massage with 50 ml glycerine and 20 drops sage oil. If this is repeated daily for the first few weeks and then weekly, rough dry skin will not have a chance to build up.

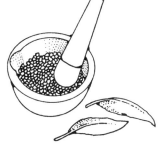

Hands

For rough, dry hands the following will provide a protective barrier.

2 tbsp beeswax
10 ml glycerine
4 drops lemon verbena or lemon oil
Melt beeswax in a double saucepan, add glycerine and oil and allow to set. A very minute amount will give hands protection. One teaspoon of zinc cream can be added to the melted beeswax for an extra booster.

Washing-up water and hard work take their toll on the hands and fingers, particularly the fingernails. The following oils help to prevent, and at the same time to heal, any dry, torn or damaged skin:

5 ml olive oil
4 drops balsam oil
4 drops sandalwood oil
2 drops Neroli oil
10 ml glycerine
Mix all the ingredients together. Massage into the cuticle region and fingers. A couple of drops rubbed into hands will help keep them soft.

Patchouli Oil for Hands and Nails
50 ml glycerine
2 gelatine capsules
12 drops patchouli oil
Mix all the ingredients together and apply after bathing or washing up.

For stains and keeping hands soft, cut slices of lemon and rub over fingers. If you are a smoker this will help remove nicotine stains.

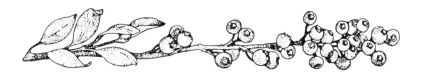

Honey and Glycerine for Hands and Face
2 tbsp beeswax
10 ml anhydrous lanolin
5 ml glycerine
2 tsp honey
1 drop benzoin
2 drops myrrh oil
In a double saucepan melt beeswax and lanolin. Add honey and stir gently until all the ingredients have dissolved. Add remaining ingredients, allow to cool in a jar that may be sealed. Use as often as hands require it.

For warts, apply a drop of thuja oil, or massage thuja cream onto them. As a lot of people suffer from warts on the hands, 2 drops of thuja oil may be added to the fore-mentioned recipe.

Massage Oil for Arthritic Hands
10 drops sassafras oil
5 drops wintergreen oil
5 drops juniper oil
20 ml cod liver oil
30 ml almond oil
Mix all the ingredients together, massaging well into fingers and joints. Wrap a hot towel compress around hands. Repeat this three to four times daily.

For those who may be suffering from any inflammatory illness such as tennis elbow this recipe is well worth trying:

Arthritis and Rheumatism Oil
50 ml castor oil
10 drops oil of wintergreen
2 cod liver oil capsules
2 drops rosemary oil
2 drops oil of juniper
Mix all the ingredients together, shake well and apply with hot compresses to affected areas. Repeat four to six times daily. To add the capsules, pierce with a hot needle and squeeze contents into oil. The odour will be camouflaged by the oil of wintergreen.

If you have had the unfortunate problem of a broken or injured bone in the hands or feet, nothing works as well as comfrey. Pick a few comfrey leaves and steep in boiling water. When cold make a compress from the liquid. Alternatively, use the leaves as a compress.

Another remedy I have tried over the years which is certainly worth a mention is cajuput oil. This oil seems to bring much relief to pain when added to some castor oil. Castor oil was one of psychic healer Edgar Cayce's favourite remedies as a cure-all, both internally and externally. I have seen it work time and time again where all else fails. I like to follow the use of it with a hot compress.

Olive oil also has a soothing and healing action. It is used as a base for many soaps, lotions and creams.

Talcs and Oils to Use as Deodorants

Commercial deodorants and powders contain aluminium which is considered a congestive agent and a possible carcinogen. They may stop you from perspiring, but the body needs to sweat to release toxins and by closing off the sweat glands with caked-on deodorants we are not allowing our bodies to perform a natural cleansing process. We are possibly doing even more damage: the incidence of lymphatic disease is steadily increasing. It is easy to make your own body talc or oil without any of the harmful chemicals.

A great oil for keeping perspiration odours away is to add 2 drops of lemon grass oil and 2 drops of lavender oil to 10 ml of glycerine. Massage a few drops under arms and on wrists. A never-fail deodorant used by many Arabs to sweeten stale perspiration on mattresses and pillows is patchouli oil. A combination of patchouli oil, lemon grass and lavender in equal portions makes a very successful antiseptic. These ingredients can be placed in a little water and used from an atomiser. Although oil and water do not emulsify, the fragrance, and particles of oil, will be dispersed. Alternatively, combine it with 25 ml apricot kernel oil and massage into underarm area.

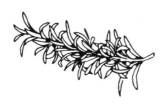

Oriental Body Talc

225 g (8 oz) starch or rice flour
125 g (4 oz) orris root powder
5 drops sandalwood oil
5 drops patchouli oil
2 drops myrrh oil
2 drops frankincense oil

Mix the ingredients together. This leaves a delightful spicy oriental fragrance and helps to absorb body moisture. The starch does not make you feel sticky and starched, but absorbs perspiration.

Lavender Deodorant

10 drops lavender oil
5 drops cinnamon oil
50 ml witch hazel

Mix ingredients and allow to stand in a cool, quiet place for two weeks — shake occasionally. Place in an atomiser and use as often as required.

or

½ cup lavender flowers
½ cup rose petals
pure alcohol or vodka

Steep flowers and petals in vodka for 3 weeks. Strain and use in a sprayer or atomiser.

Violet and Rose Body Talc

225 g (8 oz) starch or rice flour
125 g (4 oz) finely ground orris root powder
10 drops violet oil
4 drops rose oil
2 drops lavender oil

Mix all the ingredients together and place in a container with a puff or a shaker. This serves as both a talc and a body deodorant.

For the Pregnant Lady

The following 'recipes' are beneficial both before and after pregnancy. Pamper yourself; both baby and you will benefit. During pregnancy stretch marks can be a little worrying and because they look unpleasant it can bring on stress and worry for some at a time when the mind should be trouble-free.

50 ml sesame oil
10 drops geranium oil
15 drops ylang-ylang oil
10 drops lavender oil
Combine all of the oils and massage into the breasts, stomach and thighs; alternatively 25 to 30 drops may be added to your bath.

After a busy day, when you need to stop and relax, the following remedy will help you do just that.

50 ml sesame or apricot oil
15 drops lavender oil
1 drop geranium oil
8 drops sandalwood oil
Combine the oils and either add to your bath or massage directly onto skin.

Nipple Massage Oil
10 ml sweet almond oil or apricot kernel oil
1 drop rose oil
Combine the oils and massage in daily during pregnancy and before and after feeding. Massage well with clean fingers; do not worry about baby getting the fragrance when suckling, as it will not be harmful in any way. It certainly will prevent dry or cracked nipples that can bleed and become extremely painful, often going against mother's desire to feed the baby, as she has to stop.

Mastitis Oil Compress
1 pint cold lavender water
1 drop geranium oil
2 drops rose oil
Add oils to the lavender water and place in a large glass bowl; with a flannel, soak thoroughly and apply to breast area. Repeat several times daily.

For tired and aching legs, try the following:

50 ml sesame oil
20 drops lavender oil
10 drops rosemary oil
Combine the oils and massage in an upward motion over the whole leg and thigh region.

If your feet are tired, aching and carrying too much fluid, add 10 drops of juniper oil to a large dish (big enough to soak feet in) of water. Add 10 drops of the above mixture and soak feet for 10 minutes. Then massage and place feet up on a pillow, while you lie down and relax.

Perineum Healing Oil
2 drops pine oil
2 drops cypress oil
3 drops lavender oil
Add the oils to a very shallow bath. This is wonderful to use after having had a baby and tenderness due to the birth or stitches have made it a little uncomfortable to get around. The lavender, due to its antiseptic qualities, keeps infection away during the healing phase.

During those long hours of labour, to assist and make life a little easier on both mother and baby, I find the following massage oil very effective. Buy some cramp bark *(Viburnum opulus)* from a herbalist, about 15 g (½ oz) being sufficient; cut it into small pieces and pour boiling water, about 1 pint, over bark. Cool and strain after 1 hour. Soak a flannel and compress onto the womb, followed by a massage oil made with the following: 15 drops sage oil, 6 drops rose oil, and 6 drops ylang-ylang. Mix together all the ingredients into 50 ml apricot kernel oil and massage from breast to pubic region. This one is ideal for your partner to help you with. If you have an understanding doctor, he may allow you to use the oil whilst you are in hospital.

Colds and Respiratory Problems

For children or adults who have head colds or respiratory problems, try placing a couple of drops of eucalyptus oil on a piece of cloth or a hanky and place it inside the pillow case. To 25 ml castor oil add 1 drop of eucalyptus oil and massage the chest and lung region, sinus and forehead area with the massage lotion. I often put a drop of the massage solution on each nostril and my children now ask for it if they have a stuffy nose.

A word of warning: if you or your children are on homeopathic treatment, do not use the eucalyptus oil as it will counteract your treatment. Even washing your garments in eucalyptus will counteract homeopathic treatment, as will toothpaste, cigarettes and coffee.

Never use the oils on very young children; use an infusion of the herb instead.

One drop of camphor taken internally with a few grains of sugar, three times a day, will help knock a cold before it takes over. Camphor recently has become a prescription product, so its availability is somewhat limited.

Constipation

Constipation is something that happens to both young and old, generally due to either bad diet or lack of fibre in the diet. Massaging the feet and body with the following has helped many who suffer from constipation: to 50 ml apricot kernel oil, add 25 drops marjoram oil and 8 drops rose oil.

According to aromatherapy, essential oils have the ability to influence the mind, emotions and spirit, as well as the body. The following table lists various human moods and emotions, and the oils which can be used to treat them, restoring inner equilibrium.

EMOTION/MOOD	ESSENTIAL OIL
Anger/hatred	Chamomile, ylang-ylang, melissa, jasmine, rose
Exhaustion	Lavender, patchouli, myrrh, rose
Grief	Rose, hyssop, jasmine, mugwort
Impatience/irritability	Chamomile, lavender, frankincense, carnation
Indecision/indifference	Basil, patchouli, peppermint, cypress, jasmine
Jealousy/resentment	Rose, jasmine

Shyness	Jasmine, carnation, melissa, mugwort
Panic/hysteria	Chamomile, ylang-ylang, jasmine, Neroli, lavender, juniper
Shock	Neroli, lavender, melissa
Suspicion	Lavender, jasmine

Making Your Own Perfumes

Perfumes and toilet waters are either simple or compound. The former are called extracts or essences and the latter bouquets. As most of the language of the perfumer is French, this unfortunately has led to many mistakes in classification, and the terms *extraits, esprits, eaux* and *parfumes* are very loosely applied. Most materials for making perfumes and toilet waters come from the vegetable kingdom, with the exception of ambergris, civet and musk.

Ambergris is an opaque, waxy substance found floating on the sea and in the intestines of sperm whales. It has a fragrant musky odour when warmed. Its use has decreased since the whale has become an endangered species; the fragrance can now be synthesised.

Civet is a secretion from the gland beneath the tail of the civet cat. It has a strong, almost overpowering, musk-like smell, and is often used as a fixative.

Musk comes from the male musk deer, found in the Himalayan Mountains. It is a glandular secretion and is highly regarded by many Asian people as an aphrodisiac. Just as ambergris is seldom used today in order to preserve the whale populations, so musk is rarely used and is instead synthesised for fear of the deer becoming extinct.

The odours of plants reside in the roots, as in the iris and vitivert (or vetiver); the stem or wood, as in cedar and sandalwood; the leaves, as in mint, eucalyptus, patchouli and thyme; the flower, as in roses and violets; the seeds, as in the tonquin bean and caraway, and in bark, as in cinnamon.

Some citrus fruit trees yield aromatic oils; for example the oil of Neroli is obtained from the petals of *Citrus aurantium* (bitter orange), and from the rind of the fruit we obtain an essential oil of orange often called Portugal. From the leaves, on the other hand, we obtain petigrain oil. An orange tree is an invaluable asset to the operative perfumer!

The fragrances or odours of plants come, in almost every case, from a volatile oil, either contained in sacs or small vessels within them, or generated from time to time within them during their life span, as when in blossom.

Using a shallow dish, pick rose petals or flowers that you wish to use, after the morning dew has settled and before the sun is too hot. Leave the petals or flowers undisturbed for three to five days, covered with rainwater. You will then find an oily film over the top of the water – this is the essential oil. Very carefully scoop the oil out and place the tiny droplets into small glass bottles (These can be purchased cheaply from most chemists); leave uncorked until all water that may have been scooped up with the oil has completely evaporated. You may find you only have a minimal amount of volatile oil but one or two drops will render a sufficiently strong fragrance and will last for a long time. This is generally called an 'otto of roses' or an 'otto of essence'.

Some plants exude, by incision, odoriferous gums such as benzoin and myrrh; others, by the same method, give us what we call balsams, a mixture of an odorous oil and an inodorous gum. These balsams are often boiled in water for a long time, strained and boiled again until they reach the consistency of treacle. Today they are sometimes used in soap and in some cosmetics.

The odours of flowers are generally secreted during the day in the sunshine, but there are some which yield no odour in the day but become very fragrant in the evening, such as the cymbidium and catasetum. To yield large quantities of ottos (essential oils) you would need something of the following to produce the oils:

– orange peel: 4.5 kg (10 lb) produces 28 g (1 oz) oil;
– dry marjoram: 9 kg (20 lb) produces 85 g (3 oz) oil;
– fresh marjoram: 45 kg (100 lb) produces 85 g (3 oz) oil;
– patchouli herb: 50 kg (112 lb) produces 800 g (28 oz) oil;
– vetivert root: 50 kg (112 lb) produces 425 g (15 oz) oil.

The processes generally used for extracting perfumes from plants may be divided into four categories:

- expression,
- distillation,
- maceration,
- absorption.

Expression is only used where the plant has a prolific amount of volatile or essential oil, as in the outer peel of the orange, lemon and lime. One method of expression is to place the part containing the odoriferous principle in a cloth bag or press and, by force, to squeeze the oils out. The oils expressed contain water which was expelled at the same time, and by leaving it in a place where it will not be disturbed, the water and oil will separate; the oil is then poured and filtered.

Distillation involves placing the part of the plant containing the vital principle in a glass pan to which a dome lid is fitted, terminating with a pipe that is twisted corkscrew fashion and fixed in a bucket, with the end peeping out like a tap on a barrel. The water in the still is boiled. Having no other exit, the steam passes through the coiled pipe, which being surrounded with cold water in the bucket, condenses the vapour before it can arrive at the tap. The steam causes the volatile oil or perfume to rise, and is liquefied at the same time. After standing for a time, the liquids separate into two portions and are then divided, thus procuring the volatile oil.

Maceration is used for roses and many other flowers and in the making of what are known as pomades. A certain amount of odour-less vegetable oil is placed in a glass or ceramic pan and heated to around 65° Celsius. The flowers, having been carefully picked, are placed in the oil, and the heat ruptures the sacs allowing the oils to disperse into the vegetable oil. Lard and salt are used for this method also, but I prefer the vegetable oil which tends to have an affinity with the volatile oils. The oil is strained, returned to the pan and repeated several times, sometimes up to fifteen or twenty times, until the oil has the desired odour. The orange, rose and cassie compounds are principally prepared by this method. Violets *rézéda* pomades, and oils are also initially prepared this way and then finished by the absorption method.

Absorption, or enfleurage, yields not only the most exquisite essence indirectly, but also a lot of those fine pomades known as 'French pomatums' (much admired for their strength of fragrance) together with 'French oils', equally perfumed. The odours of some flowers are so delicate and volatile that the heat required in the previously mentioned processes would greatly modify, if not entirely spoil them. Absorption is therefore conducted without applying heat.

You will need square frames, about 3 inches deep, with a glass bottom 2 feet wide and 3 feet long. Over the glass, a layer of lard or pure fat is spread with a spatula. Flower buds are sprinkled over this and left for 12 to 72 hours. The flower buds are then replaced by fresh ones and this is repeated until the fat or oil is heavily perfumed. This oil may be made into creams and lotions, giving them the fragrance you desire.

To make an extract from the perfumed fat, you will require some odourless pure alcohol. Place the pomade (this is what the perfumed fat is called) into a glass bottle and pour in four quantities of alcohol to one of the pomade (for example, 10 ml of pomade to 40 ml of pure spirit). Leave to steep for 12 weeks and then skim fat off top or strain through cotton wool.

An alternative to making an extract is to use apricot kernel oil. Soak large pieces of cotton wool in oil and lay on sheets of plastic on your glass trays. Pick flowers fresh and lay on cotton wool; place second tray on top and repeat action until several trays are stacked on top of each other. A little salt (optional) may be sprinkled on the flowers. Change flowers every 2 to 3 days, ensuring cotton wool is still full of apricot oil. When the fragrance is right, squeeze oil out of cotton wool and it should be impregnated with the desired fragrance.

One of the first requisites in the manufacture of good perfumes is pure alcohol. Be sure when purchasing that it is free from an odour of any kind, as this will greatly affect the quality of the perfume. Vodka may be used for this purpose, but may need to stand for a few weeks before straining through muslin.

Essential oils can be the most fragrant room fresheners. Place 6 drops of your favourite oil into 200 ml water, using an atomiser spray; shake before use. Remember that oil and water do not mix, but they will disperse sufficiently to provide a fragrance. Spray on the backs of chairs and on pillows. Alternatively, place a couple of drops onto a radiator, candlestick or light bulb that, when turned on, will heat the oil and let the fragrance through. (Never, never put the mixture onto a light bulb that has been switched on, as it will explode and frighten your socks off!) This method of creating a room fragrance is effective for setting a mood for a party or a romantic evening.

Pennyroyal spray applied in the same way is an antidote for those nasty fleas. If your cat or dog is having problems with fleas, soak a ribbon or piece of string in pennyroyal oil and place it loosely around the animal's neck. Within 24 hours there should be no trace of fleas. Repeat this every 2 or 3 weeks.

Another way of treating fleas on your animals is to add a few drops of pennyroyal oil directly onto the coat and massage it in, being sure to include the gland area around the ears or where the collar sits, and it will be absorbed through the bloodstream. The odour will keep those nasty biting things away.

6 HERBS AND OILS FOR BATH AND BEDTIME

Herbs and oils are wonderful to utilise in bathing – for more than just the beauty of smelling good – and in herbal pillows which help you to get adequate sleep, an important factor in skin care.

Bathing in Nature

Nothing is more relaxing, yet refreshing, calming and cleansing than a lovely warm bath. For some, a cold bath is invigorating and toning after a warm bath, as it stimulates circulation. A warm bath can have a variety of oils, herbs, salts and sachets to treat health/skin problems, or to simply make you feel wonderful and leave you tingling all over.

Those who have tried it I'm sure will agree that very little in this world feels better than a bath in Epsom salts. This salt (magnesium sulphate) is similar to that found in the hot baths of Indonesia that seem to have curative qualities as well as assisting relaxation. To a warm water bath, add 2 tablespoons of Epsom salts and stir under running water. Enjoy it!

Herb sachets are great to tie onto the tap, catching the force of the running water. A lovely fragrant and relaxing one is:

½ cup lavender flowers
½ cup chamomile flowers and leaves
½ cup oatmeal powder
½ cup rose petals
½ cup skim milk powder
Tie all the ingredients together in a muslin bag or cloth. Secure with a ribbon or string and tie onto a tap, allowing running water to run over bag. The bath will smell lovely and the fragrance will seem to cling to you with a spring freshness.

If you tend to be a little nervy and hard to get going in the morning, a bath in rosemary will stimulate and give more than just a little zip to your life. Herbs are also beneficial for businessmen who may have a heavy day ahead and need to be clear-headed, particularly if the night before was a late or disturbed one. Pick 2 cups of fresh rosemary, bruise and place it in a muslin cloth or nylon stocking, and tie this to the bath tap, allowing water to run over the herbs. It is quite an overpowering smell at first, but it does clear the head; it is also a great remedy for clogged-up noses and headache. Alternatively, rosemary oil can be purchased from your health food shop or a herbalist, and only a few drops of the oil will be necessary to obtain results.

If you suffer from tinea or athlete's foot, bathing with lavender and honey acts as an antiseptic or purifier. A few drops of lavender can be massaged into the area affected as well.

Some of the following 'recipes' require bruising and pouring hot water over herbs: infusing them, just as you would to make a cup of herbal tea. However, you should *never* boil herbs unless specified. By infusing or steeping herbs, the vital ingredient is often expelled. Always use glass or pottery; aluminium and enamel containers are unsuitable. The use of muslin or stocking is occasionally specified in order to prevent the herbs sticking to your body; otherwise when you get out of your bath, it will look as though you have been tarred and feathered.

People in ancient Greece, Rome and Egypt used to bathe in milk and honey and even though it is a little extravagant, it is worth every cent. For this Isis bath you will need the following:

Isis Milk and Honey Bath
1 kg pure honey
100 g sea salt
100 g Epsom salts
 ½ kg skim milk powder
Dissolve the sea and Epsom salts in a saucepan of warm water and put into bath. Make skim milk powder mixture with boiling water to 3 litres, add honey and dissolve. Pour into bath and relax. Your skin will feel like silk.

Sea Salt Bath
This can be done in two ways. The first is by taking a handful of sea salt and rubbing it over the body, avoiding the eyes and face. Rinse off in bath or shower and then have a delicious oil bath with:
20 drops sesame oil
20 drops apricot oil
2 drops lavender oil
Mix and run into the bath.
The second way is by adding ½ cup sea salt into the bath.

Ivy Bath

2 cups fresh ivy leaves
1 cup lemon verbena
Bruise and steep with boiled water for 2 hours both the ivy and lemon verbena. Run bath, strain infusion and add under running water to disperse. A loofah sponge is ideal here for cellulite on the legs: place the leaves you have steeped in an old nylon stocking and secure with a rubber band, soap up the loofah and massage alternately with loofah and leaves.

Lavender and Honey Bath

1 cup dried lavender flowers
½ cup honey
1 tbsp sage leaves (bruised)
1 tbsp pine needles (bruised)
Pour boiling water over herbs; dissolve honey into this, strain and pour into bath. The herbs may then be tied into a bag and placed in bath. An oil-based shampoo may be used on the lavender bag to clean the body and feet.

If you or your children are ever plagued by mosquito bites or skin irritations, nothing is more soothing and relaxing than a chamomile bath. Using the flowers of the plant, either fresh or dried, steep for an hour, then pour solution into bath and relax. If your children have problems going to sleep at night, this may also assist in relaxing them.

A young patient of mine with a case of eczema, which made him scratch and tear at his skin, responded to a chamomile bath instantly. He also had a bottle of warm chamomile tea before being put to bed. His eczema, which was causing sleep problems, settled considerably and his sleeping pattern improved. A couple of tablespoons of elder flowers added to the chamomile mixture will make a stronger and equally calming bath. Elder flowers are great for acne on the body and face; the flowers, steeped for an hour or so, also make a wonderful skin tonic. The solution may be added to some plain yoghurt for skin disorders, being especially beneficial in this form for burns and scalds. Either the flowers or the young leaf buds may be used for this treatment. The elder plant (*Sambucus canadensis*) belongs to the honeysuckle family.

The following bathing remedy is especially for women who suffer from menstrual cramps. Lady's mantle (*Alchemilla vulgaris*) is astrin-.

gent in its properties and an infusion of the plant added to a warm bath works wonders. Alternatively, made as a strong tea, the solution can be used as an astringent or after-shave for both men and women.

Another remedy for women who have trouble with vaginal irritation and tenderness is a bath or a douche made from the root of the lily (white pond lily) plant. The root may be steeped or added to a muslin bag, made as a tea with boiling water and used as a douche daily. The results will speak for themselves. Being both demulcent and astringent, it is also well worth trying for throat irritations and as a mouth cleanser.

The thuja plant (*Thuja occidentalis*) works well as a counter-irritant in the relief of aches and pains of muscular origin. I have one of these trees at my front door, and to me it is one of the most beautiful trees I have ever seen. In herbal medicine I have seen nothing short of miracles occur when taking thuja as prescribed. Make a strong tea from the dried leaves and add to your bath after a day that may have taken its toll on muscles and fibres. You could also add some chamomile flowers and steep them with the thuja. A few teaspoons of Epsom salts will complement it when added under the running water. Relax and enjoy this bath.

For the sporting-minded people who need a good toner after sport or after showering or bathing, either of the following two remedies will be beneficial:

Muscular Oil for Bath and Body
50 ml apricot kernel oil
12 drops juniper oil
8 drops lavender oil
10 drops rosemary oil
5 drops wintergreen oil
Mix the ingredients and massage over body, or add 25 drops from the mixture into your bath. As oil and water do not mix, the oil in the bath clings to the body and the effect is a satin, silky feeling when you dry yourself.

Bathing and Headache Oil
20 drops rosemary oil
10 drops chamomile oil
50 ml apricot kernel oil
Mix and shake thoroughly. Massage a few drops into forehead and

temple area. Alternatively use 2 drops rosemary oil and 2 drops chamomile oil in your bath when you are feeling a little on edge and your head and body don't seem to belong together.

Many people comment on how drying a bath can be to their skin and I agree with them. But you can still soak up many an enjoyable bath either by bathing with beautiful oils added, or by using aromatic oils after your bath. In the latter case, the oils may be made into a variety of combinations using, for example, apricot kernel oil as a base for your own massage oils and bath oils.

Fragrant After-Bath Oil

I make a lovely essential oil to apply after having had a bath and before retiring:

30 ml apricot oil
20 ml jojoba oil
20 drops patchouli oil
2 drops sandalwood oil

Place 3 or 4 drops on legs, stomach and arms and massage lightly over the skin. This leaves a light but musky smell. Similar mixtures can be made using any combinations of oils that you desire.

Accessories for Body Toning

Some of the tools that may assist in toning up the body are a loofah (a large vegetable gourd which assists the removal of dead cells and at the same time tones muscles and stimulates circulation), and a sea sponge (the remnants of what was once a sea creature), a necessary cleansing tool. A nylon sponge will suffice if you are unable to get a sea sponge. A bathmit that is like a glove is very easy to use. Loofahs are sometimes manufactured as bathmits but generally they are made of towelling or flannel. A body brush is a valuable tool to have, not only for exfoliating purposes, but as these brushes generally have long handles they are great for stimulating skin tone on the back. Dry brushing is an excellent way of removing dead tissue and carried out before bathing or showering it may help to clear up many congestive skin disorders, including dermatitis and eczema.

A pumice stone, made from volcanic lava, is ideal for rubbing onto the dry, rough skin on heels and elbows before soaking them in a warm bath filled with some luxurious essential oils.

A flannel or face washer is another important working item you will need in the bathroom. Whilst soaking in your bath, I recommend adding some apricot kernel oil and the contents of a vitamin E capsule to a washer, placing the washer over the face (closing the eyes before doing so), and massaging the entire face. Leave the warm face washer in place for a few seconds, then tone the skin.

If you wish to be a little extravagant, treat your hair with essential oils, wrap in a towel, prepare your face, relax in an oil bath and I guarantee you will feel as though you have been rejuvenated from head to toe.

Making Your Own Soaps

Although making soap can be time-consuming, it provides yet another way for you to treat your skin with beneficial substances.

Some soaps benefit oily skin, others are good for dry skin; with the addition of essential oils, they will have both preventive and curative qualities. Many people say that soap is no good for your skin – and this may apply to many commercial soaps – but the soaps in this section can be medicine for your skin!

The following soap is ideal for those with sensitive skin or skin that may suffer with the problem of psoriasis or eczema. Remember that the latter conditions generally come from within, but this soap will relieve their symptoms.

Castor Oil and Glycerine Soap
500 grains Castile powder
25 g (1 oz) glycerine
15 g (½ oz) castor oil
20 drops pine oil
10 drops lavender oil
In a double saucepan melt the Castile powder to a liquid. A little boiling water added at random will benefit. When all powder has been reduced to a jelly, add glycerine, castor oil and essential oils. When mixture has cooled mould into desired shape and allow to set. This recipe is for a very soft soap; it is extremely gentle on the skin and great for young skin.

Honey and Milk Soap

1 kg Castile soap, grated or powdered
3 tablespoons milk powder
250 g pure honey
100 ml glycerine
5 ml powdered borax
2 drops geranium oil
2 drops rose oil

Place the shavings or soap powder into a glass or porcelain bowl. Mix the powdered milk in sufficient boiling water to cover the soap. Place the bowl in a double saucepan and stir until it has melted. Mix the honey, glycerine and borax and stir through the soap and milk thoroughly. Add the essential oils and mix for 10 minutes. Place mixture into a shallow baking tray and allow to cool. When cool, cut into squares. I use many different variations of this recipe. To make an oriental smelling soap with sandalwood, bergamot and patchouli, add 2 drops of each of these oils. By adding white sand and powdered oatmeal it makes the mixture very pliable. This is great for the hands, particularly if they have been subjected to grease and grime, as it whitens the dirtiest hands. Just add enough of the combined mixture to make sandsoap balls.

All hard soaps may be reduced to a fine powder, when perfectly dry, with a mortar and pestle. After cutting the soap bar into thin shavings, dry it on a large sheet of blotting paper, outside in the sunlight. As soon as the shavings become brittle they are ready for the mortar and pestle. Using small quantities at a time, powder them finely and pass the powder through a fine sieve, keeping any lumps to be sieved once more. When you have reduced to a fine powder all the shavings, place them in an airtight container until needed. Use only fine quality soap – palm oil soap, for example – for the best results. But do not use highly perfumed soaps, as you can add your own special fragrance or oil.

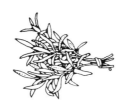

Lavender Oil Antiseptic Soap
2 cups dried lavender flowers
1 kg (2 lb) fine powdered Castile soap
40 drops lavender oil
5 g powdered orris root powder
50 ml glycerine
Powder the lavender flowers in a mortar or coffee grinder. Mix soap, lavender powder and orris root powder together, cover with boiling water and stand in a double saucepan until soap is dissolved. Add lavender oil and glycerine and set in a tray. If mixture appears to be too soft, a little rosin powder can be added, as can salt. The rosin will give the mixture a yellow colour. A few drops of cochineal may be added to give a red or pink colour.

To make a pumice stone soap, dissolve coconut oil soap in a small quantity of water and run it into moulds. Add half its weight of powdered pumice stone and stir the whole until it sets. This is a great soap for the mechanic.

To make transparent soap, the best method is the one known as the 'alcohol process', which consists of dissolving ordinary, good opaque soap, made from tallow, lard and other fats and oils, in boiling alcohol and subsequently evaporating the solvent, leaving the soap in a more or less transparent condition. By this process, any carbonate of the alkali, sulphate of sodium and any other impurities present in the original soap, are entirely eliminated in the finished product, as these substances are insoluble in the strong alcohol. The solution of soap, which is at first reduced to shavings and dried as thoroughly as possible, is placed in a double saucepan until all the soap has dissolved. The mixture is then placed in another vessel, in which alcohol has been distilled off and condensed. The residue of hot soap is withdrawn and is then placed in a suitable frame to set. After cutting the soap, which is usually muddy in appearance, it is exposed for some time to warm air to evaporate the remaining traces of alcohol and water, during which time it becomes clear and transparent. By being kept for a long time, and through exposure to air, the soap darkens in colour, acquiring a rich amber tint. The addition of glycerine generally improves the quality of the soap.

You can make variations of these soaps, forming them in whatever shape you wish: they make wonderful gifts to put in a basket with a potpourri. The quantities may be changed depending on the amount you wish to make.

Bubble bath liquid is popular with children, and this recipe is a winner:

1 cake of white Castile soap
50 ml glycerine
distilled water or rainwater
Cut the soap into thin pieces, dry and powder finely, place in a litre bottle and fill the bottle with the distilled water; shake well, until all the soap has been saturated into a solution. Leave to stand for a few minutes and if the solution settles, you are ready for the next step. If the solution does not settle, pour off 90 per cent of the water and replace with fresh distilled water and shake well as before. The glycerine should be added when the water finally clears. If you wish to fragrance the bubble bath, add a few drops of your favourite essential oil; for example, chamomile.

Herbal Pillows

Adequate rest and sleep is of course vital to the maintenance of healthy skin. Missing your required amount of sleep on a regular basis will affect the skin noticeably, possibly causing specific skin disorders. Many people find herbal pillows invaluable if they suffer from insomnia, restlessness or snoring.

Insomnia Pillow
1 cup mugwort
1 cup verbena (dried)
1 cup lavender (dried)
1 cup hops (dried)
2 drops Neroli oil
2 tsp orris root powder
Making a pillow approximately 30cm (12 inches) square, place two thin layers of cotton wool or dacron of the same dimension inside. Sprinkle herbs between cotton wool or dacron and sew up pillow. Place under bed pillow, or in such a way that no little rough parts of the herbs will protrude. Crush pillow lightly to bring forth fragrance. This recipe makes 6-8 pillows.

Baby Pillow for Sleep
2 drops Neroli oil
1 cup hops
1 cup chamomile flowers
1 cup tea-tree leaves
2 tsp orris powder (fixative)
Make as for the preceding pillow. Lavender may be added to this as it is calming in its effect and smells a little more pleasant than the hops, or 2 drops of lavender oil added to the dry herbs will suffice. This also makes a great mattress for the newborn baby and costs very little. I have seen young babies slip into the 'perfect' sleeping pattern after the first introduction to the pillow.

For those people who claim 'I never snore' but the partner disagrees, the following should help stop the snoring, so that breathing can once again be restored to normal:

'Snoreless' Pillow
1 cup hops
1 cup tea-tree leaves
1 drop eucalyptus oil
2 drops Neroli oil
2 tsp orris root powder
Place dried herbs in dacron, sprinkle orris powder over and add oil. Place inside a pillow case, or alternatively make as a potpourri and leave jar uncovered next to the bed (the latter is not as effective, but it still brings results).

Herbs for pillows are often best reduced to a powder in a grinder or mortar. Mix all the herbs together, add oil and place in a sachet inside pillow. These make wonderful, economical gifts and after a good, restful night's sleep your skin will show the benefit.

7 REFLEXOLOGY: RESTORING HEALTH THROUGH THE FEET

If certain organs of the body are functioning below par, then this in turn will affect the glands, bloodstream and eventually the skin, to varying degrees. Reflexology, or zone therapy, assists in diagnosing and treating body ailments, as well as in disease prevention, and is thus a valuable tool in both corrective and preventive skin care.

It is a therapy which focuses on the reflex points in the feet, based on the fact that there are about 72000 nerve endings in each foot which connect to other parts of the body. Massage is applied to those nerve endings, when necessary, thus conveying an impulse to the organs which are not functioning correctly.

Reflexology dates back to the ancient Egyptians, and to China and India over 5000 years ago. As the saying goes, everything that works, and contains the truth, will survive the test of time. Herbal remedies, acupuncture, massage and many other forms of natural medicine have survived this test of time.

Reflexology helps to keep the energy of the body in harmony. Because man wears shoes and socks, and generally does very little in the way of exercising, the energy that travels through our bodies becomes congested and forms crystals that hamper this natural flow. If we were to take our shoes off and walk on a path of pebbles or stones, we would probably feel pressure and pain at the same time. yet natives of various countries who seldom wear shoes, and whose feet are therefore constantly stimulated, are generally a lot healthier than we are.

Imagine that the body is divided in half and from each toe a meridian or energy passes through to the top of the head, and likewise from the fingers. This gives us five main energy flows – or zones – on either side of the body.

Foot Massage

I have consistently checked and researched the principles of reflexology, and its accuracy and results are astounding! You will find that if you press hard into the part of the foot which relates to a troubled organ, a sharp penetrating pain in the foot will result. This pain will feel as if a needle or sharp instrument is being pushed into that part of the foot. In this way, deep digital rotary massage applied on the foot easily finds trouble spots and the organ concerned.

When this massage is first applied, it is important that the troubled areas are not over-stimulated at first. It is surprising how sore some of these spots can become. If you are performing reflexology on yourself, you may find the use of a zone roller a help. This can be made with a large ball-bearing castor, the type that is used on the legs of chairs or tables. This castor is sunk into a block of thick wood and the foot is pressed and rotated on top of the ball bearing, which will rotate with the movements of the foot. A golf ball will serve the same purpose, or even a small smooth pebble will help to break down the crystallisation that gathers around the nerve endings in the feet. It is this crystal that causes such pain when it is pushed into the sheaths of the nerves concerned.

Zone therapy or reflexology is wonderful in relieving glandular ailments. The importance of glands is well known: if one gland malfunctions, we get an imbalance in the whole of the endocrine system that can produce tremendous upsets throughout the whole of the body.

Miraculous results can be achieved by giving compression massage to the reflex of the pituitary gland, the reflex which is found in the centre of the ball of each big toe. The location of this gland is at the base of the brain, therefore any congestion in the neck will retard the blood supply to that gland, and will create a pathological condition. This is the cause of many breakdowns — a phobia or fear results and trivial troubles are magnified out of all proportion. It affects the chemical content and the pH of the blood, and nervous hypertension increases, thus producing a pathological residue into the bloodstream that must be eliminated from the body, via the organs of excretion.

All disease, whatever its name, can be classified under one heading, that is, congestion. That word or condition covers everything in the pathological field. Foot massage, applied correctly, relieves this congestion of the organ under stress, stimulating and activating that organ, and relieving the crystallised condition of the nerve endings. In this way, zone therapy safely and gently uses compression massage on painful areas of the feet to clear away diseased conditions from the body.

A condition which often indicates congestion within the body is fallen arches. As the muscular condition weakens, the complete body structure also deteriorates, shifting the position of the twenty-six bones in the foot. We then get undue pressure on some of the nerve endings in the feet, which cuts off some of the normal blood and nerve supply in the soles of the feet, thereby slowing down circulation.

This leads to the formation of chemical deposits, or morbid matter around the articulations of the feet – the condition known as fallen arches. If this condition lasts long enough we shall find trouble in other parts of the body. If, for example, this obstruction is on the nerve ending or reflex to the liver, we find this organ being robbed of some of its blood supply, thus affecting its normal functions. Naturally, the longer the condition lasts, the longer it takes to correct it.

But even in cases where the feet appear to be in perfect condition, tender areas are often found on the soles. This can be caused by some organ, or part of the body, which is not functioning as it should and is unable to contract and relax as it would normally. This means that the circulation to the part concerned is not strong enough to keep the nerve endings free from the formation of crystals, which in turn causes pain in the corresponding foot zone when pressed.

A lesion in any part of the spine is bound to interfere with normal circulation and reduce contraction and relaxation of the part which is depending upon particular nerves for its blood supply. If this is the case, we then find tenderness in the spinal reflex zones in the feet. Those zones are situated in the inside border of each foot, just above the 'waist line' (smallest part) of the foot. This is a good adjunct therapy for osteopathy. If we study the nervous system, we can see at a glance how dependent it is on the spine for its blood supply. Therefore, the slightest undue pressure on the spine will interfere with the contracting and relaxing process, necessary to keep the nerve endings to the feet and the corresponding part of the body free from crystalline deposits.

By referring to a reflexology chart of the feet, you can diagnose your own ailments: apply firm pressure with your thumbs to the feet, and you will soon pick out the body part that is sending out the danger signal. You will be quite surprised at the tenderness or even pain associated with some of the trouble spots, even when you have not been conscious of any pain there before. If massaging, be gentle if the part is tender, working only a few minutes each day, until the desired benefits are attained.

Most of us have heard the saying 'My feet are killing me!' Often when this is the case, the whole body feels ill. Yet we usually do not investigate whether there is any connection between this pain in the feet and our poor physical condition!

The hands also have 'zones' which relate to other parts of the body.

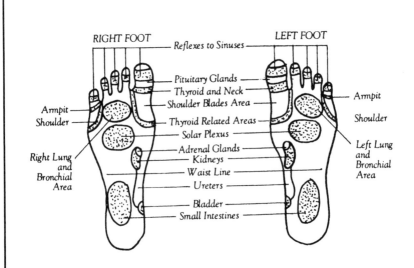

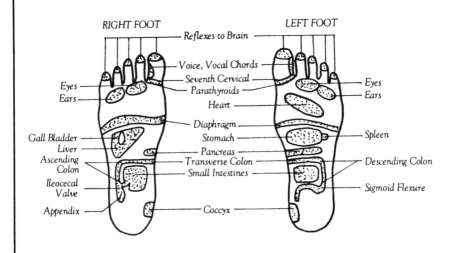

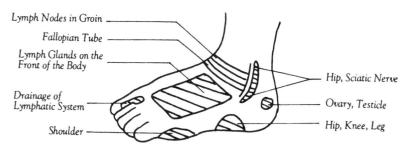

LEFT FOOT OUTSIDE
The same reflexes are on the right foot outside

Lymph Nodes in Groin

Fallopian Tube

Lymph Glands on the
Front of the Body

Drainage of
Lymphatic System

Shoulder

Hip, Sciatic Nerve

Ovary, Testicle

Hip, Knee, Leg

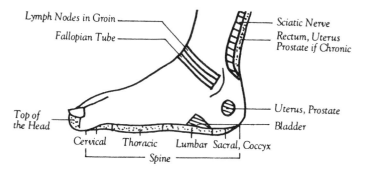

RIGHT FOOT INSIDE
The same reflexes are on the left foot inside

Lymph Nodes in Groin

Fallopian Tube

Sciatic Nerve

Rectum, Uterus
Prostate if Chronic

Top of
the Head

Uterus, Prostate

Bladder

Cervical   Thoracic   Lumbar   Sacral, Coccyx

Spine

Recently, I treated a friend who is a drummer in a rock band. His hands were sore and sensitive, but after 10 minutes of firm massage to the zones on each hand, he felt 'better all over'. People who over-exert the hands are often more prone to arthritic tendencies later in life. By massaging regularly, congestion will not have a chance to take place, preventing the onset of rheumatism, arthritis, eczema and disease that plagues so many of us, and not only in later life. People who over-exert their hands due to the nature of their work should massage their feet and hands weekly.

Treating with Reflexology

When conducting foot massage, you will soon be able to judge – by the amount of pain present – the severity of the condition you are dealing with. Generally, the older the patient, the larger the crystals under the zone will be, and naturally they will cause more pain. As we massage those crystals, we gradually break them down and cause small particles to be driven into the muscle tissue. It is usually the case that the second, third and fourth treatments are more painful, owing to this fact. At each treatment we are causing an acceleration of the circulation of the blood through the parts affected, thereby increasing the vitality and endurance of the person.

Use your own discretion as to the length of time you spend on each area of the foot, but do not over-stimulate or cause too much pain. Remember, you are stimulating the circulation, which in turn raises the body's vitality, helping to throw off the poisons that have been causing the trouble. The more toxic material the blood contains, the more severe the reaction will be. Often the reaction is a severe cold, so do not be alarmed if this healing crisis manifests itself. It shows that the body is eliminating toxic waste through another channel.

Some people are very sensitive and find it hard to relax while you massage. Start gently and build up over a period of several weeks, and you will find that the problem areas do not create so much discomfort.

Massage in a forward rotary motion, using the exterior corner of the thumb rather than the ball of the thumb. Let the pressure be firm and even, but not too great to start with. Increase the pressure gradually. Always be guided by the expression on the face of the person being treated. Make sure that they are warm and comfortable, so that they can receive the full benefits of the treatment.

Remember to keep the finger nails short and the hands clean. If you are practising reflexology on someone else, they may accuse you of jabbing them with your nail as the pressure can sometimes feel like that.

Locating the Reflexes

Sit facing the person you wish to treat, take the left foot in your right hand, holding the foot firmly. With the thumb and first finger of the left hand, grasp the smallest part of the foot, generally about halfway along the sole. This is called the 'waist line' of the foot. The reflexes to the various organs situated above the body waistline are located above this area of the foot. Those organs that are wholly situated on the left side of the body only have a reflex on the left foot and vice versa. Those organs we find on both sides of the body, such as the lungs, have reflex zones on both feet. (Remember that the lungs have a strong bearing, in many ways, on your skin.)

The **heart** is reflected only on the left foot, the **liver** on the right foot, and the **large intestine** takes up a generous portion on both feet, due to the momentous job it does. The reflex for the **ascending colon** is on the right foot, as is the right half of the **transverse colon**, as it crosses the abdomen from right to left, just below the liver reflex under the waist line. It then crosses over to the left foot, where it becomes the **descending colon**, and runs down the outside of the left foot.

The **small intestine** is found in the centre of the large intestine. You can therefore, by compression massage, find out approximately which part of the intestine is causing trouble, thus allowing diagnosis of problems such as constipation, which often results in irritability and headaches, and allows vast amounts of toxins to enter the bloodstream, once again affecting our skin, our behaviour and our breath.

The **appendix** is at the lower border of the ascending colon on the righthand side, so the reflex for this is on the right foot just above the heel. If you come across what is called a 'grumbling appendix', zone therapy will be invaluable. Indeed it soon clears up the congestion and many an appendix has been saved for its owner simply by reflexology massage.

The **stomach** is located just above the waist line of the foot, in the first, second, third and fourth zones in the left foot. In an acute attack of gastric influenza, compression massage to the stomach reflexes is invaluable and will cut short such attacks.

Each **kidney** comes into the third zone of each foot, just above the waist. The **gall bladder**, attached to the liver, has its reflex in the right foot, a little under the ball of the foot.

The **lungs and bronchial tubes** are found on both sides of the body; consequently their reflexes occur on both feet, just below the base of the toes. In pneumonia, compression massage for the lung reflexes will render great relief.

The **eyes** have their reflexes between the first, second and third toes and also at the base of the second and third toes on both feet. Both feet need treatment. A number of the patients I see have eye complaints, some serious, some being merely astigmatism or a slight flattening of the eyeball. While some cases are not able to benefit greatly from reflexology, others respond well, so it is well worth trying for all eye complaints.

The reflexes of the **ears** are between and at the base of the third and fourth toes. Reflexology can do wonders for the ears. Deafness, like blindness, can be caused by many conditions, some of which are outside the scope of any therapy, but in some cases zone therapy has given wonderful results. This, of course, depends on the cause, but it is worth a serious trial. Always use zone therapy in catarrhal deafness.

Nasal catarrh and sinus problems are caused, as usual, by congestion; by massaging daily or weekly the correct reflex, the cause can be removed, rather than suppressed (as in most other forms of treatment). The reflexes are just below the tips of the toes on each toe. Both feet and both sides of the toes must be massaged. Massaging these points is also ideal for hay fever sufferers. Try it before you judge it and be patient!

The **pituitary gland** is considered to be one of the most important in the ductless group. If we can have it functioning correctly we shall automatically put right many of the secondary complaints in the body, so I advise you when practising zone work to start on the reflex to this gland, which is found in the ball of each big toe. This gland controls height, both large and small. An unusual condition known as acromegaly, where the tongue, nose, hands and feet are excessively large, is caused by an imbalance of the pituitary gland. Headaches are often caused by this gland. Nervousness and lack of confidence in oneself are also conditions attributed to this gland. I have found it to be of great value for suppressed menses and menopause. This will also affect the other glands in the body, creating symptoms of tender spots in other gland areas. Insomnia often will respond after this gland has settled, and sleepful nights replace sleepless ones!

The **thyroid gland** has two lobes, situated one on each side of the trachea. They are connected by an isthmus stretching across the front of the neck. The cavities of the thyroid gland are filled with an iodine material, the active principle which keeps us in tune with our surroundings. This gland works closely in harmony with other ductless glands. An imbalance here will affect other glands and vice versa. Our moods and our skin will quickly show the problem outwardly if nothing has been detected inwardly.

The **ovaries** have a very close relationship with the thyroid gland, so if we find the thyroid out of condition, we shall very likely find some trouble in the ovaries. Therefore, always treat both areas when treating thyroid or ovaries. You will find the point for the ovaries at the back of the ankle. The thyroid and neck points are at the base of the big toes of each foot.

The **pancreas** is a very large, important gland, having a great deal to do with the metabolism of the body. It supplies lymph and insulin to the blood. The set of glands which are antagonistic to this one are the adrenals. The adrenals secrete adrenalin, which raises the sugar content of the blood. Insulin, on the other hand, whether administered by the pancreas or artificially, will lower the sugar in the blood. The ductless system is of primary importance to the whole of the body and its related health. The point for the pancreas is found on the left foot around the waist line region. You will find tenderness in this area if you are diabetic.

Treating these points on the feet assists in skin care by correcting imbalances within; the body's rejuvenation will be reflected in a much healthier skin.

If one drop of an essential oil is used on the reflex of a particular organ, treatment will be considerably enhanced. I call this 'Aromaology'. Some important facts to be aware of are:

- Be relaxed yourself, or your patient will feel uneasy.
- Perform the treatment in a clean, warm room.
- Select a comfortable chair for yourself.
- Select a comfortable chair or couch for your patient.
- A light hospital blanket may be used, as body heat is lost when lying still.

- Make sure the patient's clothing is loose and not restricting. (Remove jewellery, watches, etc.)
- The patient's head should be slightly elevated, so that facial expressions can be observed.
- If the patient is relaxed, the treatment will be more successful.

Some changes will be noted in patients if their diet has been heavily spiced or changes from the normal pattern, of if they have had changes in health due to the weather, for example, cold snaps, heat, winds or a latent illness that may be still brewing, or trauma and emotional disturbances. Everyone benefits from reflexology, from babies to our senior generations.

The following list indicates the oils suitable for each complaint:

Abscess	Lavender, bergamot, rose, camphor
Acidity	Rosemary, sage, chamomile, neroli
Acne	Bergamot, sandalwood, lavender, cedarwood
Allergies	Melissa, chamomile, ylang-ylang
Alopecia	Lavender, rosemary
Antiseptics	Eucalyptus, lavender, rose, myrrh, rosemary
Anxiety	Ylang-ylang, lavender, jasmine, neroli, rose
Arthritis	Cajuput, benzoin, eucalyptus, rosemary, wintergreen, lavender
Asthma	Cypress, eucalyptus, hyssop, benzoin, melissa
Bladder	Juniper, lavender, parsley, bucha, chamomile
Boils	Clary sage, lavender, chamomile
Breasts	Rose, ylang-ylang, lavender, geranium
Bronchitis	Benzoin, basil, bergamot, eucalyptus, hyssop, lavender
Catarrh	Eucalyptus, sandalwood, hyssop, frankincense, lavender
Cellulitis	Rosemary, juniper, lavender, hyssop
Circulation	Clary sage, hyssop, melissa, cypress
Colds	Basil, eucalyptus, melissa, pennyroyal
Colic	Chamomile, fennel, parsley, juniper, spearmint or peppermint

Conjunctivitis	Chamomile, rose, lavender (as a compress)
Constipation	Castor oil, rose, lavender, fennel
Cough	Black pepper, cardamom, cypress, clary sage
Cystitis	Bergamot, juniper, lavender, myrrh
Depression	Ylang-ylang, chamomile, jasmine, rose, mugwort, sandalwood
Dermatitis	Juniper, avocado, lavender, olive oil
Diabetes	Agrimony, geranium, juniper
Diarrhoea	Black pepper, chamomile, lavender, peppermint, eucalyptus
Earache	Hyssop, lavender, myrrh, cajuput
Eczema	Bergamot, chamomile, lemon grass, hyssop, hypericum, neroli, ylang-ylang
Enuresis	Cypress, ylang-ylang
Eyes	Eyebright, fennel
Fainting	Lavender, peppermint, melissa, angelica
Fevers	Peppermint, yarrow, melissa, basil
Fistula	Lavender, rose
Flatulence	Calamus, clary sage, fennel, peppermint, chamomile, garlic
Gall bladder	Chamomile, lavender, rosemary
Gingivitis	Myrrh, bergamot, sage, thyme
Gonorrhoea	Lavender, cedarwood, bergamot, cypress
Gout	Uva ursi, elder, basil, lemon grass, fennel, juniper
Haemorrhoids	Garlic, cypress, juniper, myrrh, bergamot
Halitosis	Cardamom, lavender, peppermint
Hayfever	Melissa, chamomile, rose
Headache	Lemon, lavender, melissa, mint, cardamom
Heart palpitations	Lavender, melissa, ylang-ylang, peppermint, rosemary
Hepatitis	Rosemary
Herpes	Bergamot, lemon
Hysteria	Cajuput, lavender, rosemary, rose, hyssop

Impotence	Jasmine, rose, sandalwood, ylang-ylang
Indigestion	Carraway, lavender, mint
Infections	Basil, rosemary, sage, thyme, ylang-ylang, garlic, lavender, lemon
Influenza	Garlic, elecampane, chamomile, lemon, cypress, eucalyptus, lavender, pine, neroli, rosemary, sage
Insect bites	Garlic, pennyroyal, lemon, lavender, sage, basil
Insomnia	Chamomile, lavender, neroli, rose, sandalwood, mugwort, ylang-ylang
Intestines (colitis, etc.)	Garlic, hyssop, juniper, lavender, neroli, thyme, verbena
Itching	Garlic, elecampane, cinnamon, carraway, lemon, lavender, rosemary, pennyroyal
Jaundice	Rosemary, cypress, juniper, rose
Kidney (general)	Cedarwood, clary, lavender, juniper
Nephritis	Chamomile, eucalyptus, tea-tree
Pyelitis	Cedarwood, juniper, pine
Laryngitis	Benzoin, frankincense, lemon, sandalwood, lavender
Leucorrhoea	Bergamot, clary, eucalyptus, hyssop, mugwort, elecampane
Lice	Sassafras, pennyroyal
Liver	
Chlorosis	Lavender, myrrh, cypress, rosemary
Cirrhosis	Rosemary, hyssop
Congestion	Chamomile, hyssop, cypress, rosemary, sandalwood
Lungs	Garlic, cajuput, cypress, tea-tree, fennel, clove, hyssop, pine, sage

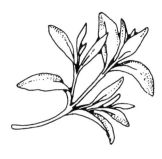

Malaria	Garlic, lemon, tea-tree, eucalyptus
Measles	Chamomile, eucalyptus, lavender, thyme
Melancholia	Lavender, ylang-ylang
Memory loss	Clove, rosemary, cardamom
Menopause	Chamomile, cypress,sage, fennel
Menorrhagia	Cypress, rose
Menstration irregularity	Clary sage, melissa, rose, clove
Dysmenorrhoea	Cypress, jasmine, rose, clary sage, lavender
Scantiness	Chamomile, clary sage, fennel, melissa, peppermint
Mental fatigue	Basil, clove, cardamom
Migraine	Basil, eucalyptus, melissa, marjoram
Nails (broken)	Lemon
Nausea	Parsley, bergamot, juniper, lavender, myrrh
Neuralgia	Chamomile, yarrow, geranium
Nosebleed	Cypress, frankincense
Obesity	Patchouli, fennel, neroli, juniper, lemon
Oedema	Juniper, myrrh, fennel
Ovaries	Cypress
Pneumonia	Camphor, angelica
Pregnancy	Clary sage, melissa, juniper, ylang-ylang
Prostate	Pine, tea-tree
Pruritis	Elecampane, chamomile, mint, lavender
Rheumatism	Garlic, cajuput, chamomile, lemon, tea-tree, pine, rosemary
Scalds	Lavender, rose
Sinusitis	Cinnamon, lemon, mugwort, neroli, rosemary
Skin	
Chapped	Lemon, benzoin, geranium
Eczema	Lavender, elecampane, cypress, violet, myrrh, sandalwood
Dry	Chamomile, geranium, jasmine, sandalwood, ylang-ylang

Oily	Bergamot, camphor, cedarwood, frankincense
Mature	Benzoin, clary, cypress, frankincense, myrrh, patchouli, jasmine, rose, mugwort
Sensitive	Chamomile, jasmine, rose, lavender, violet
Sprains	Pine, eucalyptus, tea-tree, rosemary
Throat infections	Clary, eucalyptus, lavender
Thrush	Myrrh
Tonsillitis	Bergamot, lavender
Toothache	Clove, pennyroyal, peppermint
Ulcers	
Corneal	Lavender, chamomile
Mouth	Myrrh, pennyroyal
Peptic	Chamomile, geranium
Varicose	Bergamot, lavender, castor oil
Urticaria	Chamomile
Vaginitis	Chamomile
Varicose veins	Cypress
Vertigo	Basil, chamomile, lavender
Vomitting	Chamomile, fennel, melissa, peppermint
Whooping cough	Cypress, hyssop, rosemary, tea-tree
Worms	Bergamot, chamomile, eucalyptus, fennel, hyssop, melissa, peppermint
Wounds	Benzoin, frankincense, geranium, hyssop, lavender, myrrh, patchouli

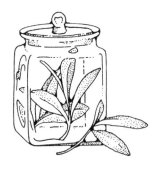

8 ACUPUNCTURE FOR THE FACE AND BODY

Acupuncturists often associate lines on the face with certain organs that may be under par. As well as reading the pulse in wrists and ankles, they observe lines on the cheeks, eyes and forehead. Using this to assist their diagnosis, acupuncturists can treat problems such as sinus, neuralgia, headaches and skin conditions.

Specific hair growth on the chin and top lip region often indicates hormonal problems; the deep furrows between our eyes are generally due to stomach and liver imbalances. This does not necessarily indicate that disease is present, but rather, that there is an energy breakdown to that part of the body, which in time could lead to disease of the body. If a person frowns constantly they are normally stressed or worried. This may be due to depression or a general feeling of being unwell. In grandmother's day the saying that a person 'is just plain liverish' meant that the liver was a little firey or heated. I have seen acupuncturists perform some great rejuvenating effects by working on a troubled organ through its relationship with certain facial lines. Mini face-lifts are also being performed by acupuncturists worldwide, with very pleasing results.

Diagnosing Through Skin Colour

The Chinese believe that the complexion refers to both the colour and state of the flesh. It is the reflection on the exterior of the state of the organs and entrails, of blood and energy. It is also the reflection on the exterior of their pathological condition.

In acupuncture, the variation of the skin's colour determines the state of emptiness or fullness of energy and blood, and will follow the progression of a disease, since the internal organs are closely linked to circulation. The deterioration of the internal organs can lead to bad circulation.

The five colours listed below correspond to the five elements system and are related to both seasons and the organs.

Green	Liver	Spring
Red	Heart	Summer
Yellow	Spleen	End of summer
White	Lungs	Autumn
Black	Kidneys	Winter

- Signs of pain are reflected by black, white and green.
- Signs of fullness are reflected by yellow and red.
- Signs of emptiness are reflected by white.

When a patient comes to an acupuncturist with red skin, it is usually caused by the following:

- heat or a congestive state of the body where elimination is insufficient;
- fever: fullness of heat in the interior body;
- a heart condition (usually signalled by a dark red face often accompanied by cold hands and feet and looseness of bowels).

When people have a yellowish colour, it generally indicates a problem with the spleen and stomach. Skin colour also varies with factors such as wind and heat. The absence of colour, when skin appears white, can indicate lack of energy, exhaustion, illness, anaemia and shock. Healthy white skin should be slightly pink. Green is the colour that appears when congestion is due to cold or the depletion of energy through pain. A green similar to the colour of grass is a sign of exhaustion of liver meridian energy. The black that appears under eyes or on the skin relates to kidney emptiness or emptiness of the blood. If an abnormal colour moves to the top of the head, it is generally a bad sign. If it moves to the bottom, it is generally good, so the Chinese have claimed for thousands of years.

Distinct colour indicates recent diseases, usually not serious, whereas indistinct colour indicates a chronic and more serious disease. Those numerous white spots that occur on the face or legs can be caused by parasitic invasion and red cheeks can mean too much fire within a certain organ.

A Chinese doctor and lecturer recently specified that the colours of the face lead to three judgements as to their cause:

- state of circulation;
- state of the nervous system;
- state of the digestive system.

The brightness of the face's colour is related to circulation. A healthy body will have a certain glow on the face and that means healthy in both mind and body. The nervous system will reflect in any green, yellow, red, white or black tones. Some people may appear to have a green colour around the mouth and nose. This indicates the heart's nerves are not in harmony. If there are patches of colour on the face, or if the lower half and upper half are of different colours, or if the right and left parts of the face are of different shades, then the cause is indigestion. If there is a burning sensation in the face then there is an imbalance in the stomach meridian.

The acupuncturist looks for all these vital signs and pulse abnormalities and treats the cause accordingly. Having disregarded acupuncture for a long time, the western world is now beginning to take seriously this ancient technique. It is well known that acupuncture involves needles that are very fine, penetrating between the pores of the skin on the surface of the body for therapeutic or pain relieving purposes. Many people do not realise that utilising needles is not the only method the acupuncturist uses to stimulate a certain meridian. Acupressure, moxibustion, iron granules and electronic methods are also used to stimulate certain points and these are a great advantage for those who 'fear' needles. I used to be one of those people, but after getting used to them, I now thoroughly enjoy a treatment and generally after the needles have been inserted, I fall asleep for half an hour. It is really very relaxing. After I have had several treatments people often comment on how much 'younger' I look.

Acupuncture to Diminish Wrinkles

When having acupuncture to reduce wrinkles, the practitioner will examine the contour of the face and determine the condition of the muscles beneath the skin, which have the function of holding the shape of the flesh. A young face has an evenly formed and firm shape because the muscles are strong and elastic. A moist, supple skin will not crease or wrinkle as easily as a dry skin (the drier the skin, the deeper the wrinkle lines will etch themselves).

The skin (both the epidermis and dermis layers) always follows its foundation, which is the muscle structure. Wherever parts of the face move then we can be sure that muscles are attached to the inner layer of skin, and these are the places where lines or wrinkles develop. If we could not move a muscle in our face, then we would not get lines. People who very rarely show emotion, whether it be tears or laughter, and who have a 'deadpan' expression constantly, may still get lines because those emotions will store within, giving congestion and stress factors.

If we sleep in a certain position we may wake up finding creases on our faces and arms. After a short while, these generally disappear as the moisture in the skin plumps them out. Over the first 25 to 30 years the muscles gradually lose their stability and firmness, the environment and pollution take their toll and moisture loss becomes apparent. In Chinese acupuncture, management of facial wrinkles must be on the muscular and energy plane, as well as restoring moisture, circulation and tone to the skin.

Pressure applied to specific acupuncture points will help relax those areas, stimulate energy flow and allow circulation back to clogged-up areas. If you use both reflexology for the feet and acupressure for the face, both poles of the body are helped with decongestion or energy blocks which may occur along any of the meridians. (Readers are advised to purchase a chart of acupuncture points for the face.)

Signs in the Lips and Teeth

Using the many signs that the body shows us, doctors look at our tongues, check our eyes and hands, press and prod, all of which assists in the diagnosis and evaluation of our general health condition. An acupuncturist reads your pulse, looks at the colour of the tongue and reads facial lines. The colour of the skin, bags under the eyes, the state of the lips, facial hair, ridges on the nails, skin blemishes and the like indicate to him any pending or current problems.

If there are marks on the upper lip, the practitioner will be looking closely at the stomach, oesophagus and pylorus. The lower lip reflects problems in the small and large intestines. If the lips seem to hang loosely this can indicate poor digestion and loss of nutrients, a bad bowel pattern and putrefaction of the bowels. So many children seem to have their mouths open constantly and this is not always because they can't breathe through their noses. This can often show an imbalance in the metabolic function which is chronically congested; lethargy, tiredness and irritability are often the first behavioural signs that are noticed. Bright red lips indicate blood pressure and respiratory problems. White lips show that anaemia or lack of oxygen could be the problem. Too many fatty acids and high cholesterol in the blood will show in dark red-blue lips.

Lines extending up and down on the lips (lipstick seems to run into these lines) indicate hormonal changes. These often begin to show when we are in our mid- to late-thirties, as our hormones change. If a young person develops lip lines it is wise to consult an acupuncturist, as it could be a sign of weakness in the reproductive areas. All these body signs are warnings that something is wearing down, needing regeneration or creating imbalances that will cause problems later on.

Your teeth show an acupuncturist a lot more than whether you brush them or not. Widely spaced teeth reveal certain characteristics of excretory and respiratory functions. The front teeth represent the thoracic area, lungs, heart and bronchial tubes. The canines represent the liver, pancreas and duodenum. The molars reflect the state of the reproductive system, intestines and kidneys.

The possible side effects from amalgam fillings are being heavily researched in America and by some of our leading dental specialists here in Australia. It is believed that small particles of mercury are expelled from these fillings into the bloodstream and that this toxic substance can create allergies and skin disorders. It is interesting to correlate recent research with the old saying 'as mad as a hatter' which began when mercury was used in the making of hats to keep them in shape; it was later discovered that mercury was absorbed through the skin, creating insanity or changing moods.

Rushing to your dentist is not the answer, nor is having all your fillings changed to porcelain. All this could allow more particles to escape during removal of the old fillings. For future dentistry, find a sympathetic dentist and he will advise you as to your needs.

Signs In and Around the Eyes

The iris is the iridologist's most valuable tool. To an acupuncturist the colour around the eyes and under them is an important diagnostic tool. Fluids that are accumulating caused by weak or overloaded kidneys will produce a blue-black colour below the eyes, as will a person under stress and in need of a peaceful sleep. The fluid bags and dark circles indicate inflammation and possible infection in the reproductive system.

A puffy brown bag, as often seen by those who indulge in excess alcohol, fats and rich living is the result of a congested or sick liver. If a person gets jaundice or hepatitis, a disease of the liver, the whites of the eyes go yellow. Often when I give my patients a liver clean-out, the first remark is 'My eyes feel so much better, and they seem to have that sparkle back again'. Headaches and skin disorders seem to disappear and good bowel habits are re-established once more. The skin again shows that healthy glow.

People who constantly blink or have dilated pupils or eyes that never seem to keep still, are generally under a lot of nervous stress. The nervous system in fact ends at the eyes, reminding us of the saying that they are a mirror to the soul. Those who have a dark circle surrounding the eyes may find that it is their nervous system crying out. As mentioned earlier, the goings-on inside will reflect on the outside, so sometimes instead of cleansing the face we should begin by cleaning up the inside – and just watch the eyes and skin change. !

Signs in the Skin

When our bodies are in a state of imbalance the skin is quite often the first place to send out a visible signal. The pimples and blemishes that appear are simply a warning that the body is out of harmony. If pimples appear on your back the lungs and kidneys could be at fault; if on the chest, the lungs and heart meridians; if on the forehead, the intestines could be sluggish; if on the cheeks, the lungs could be over-loaded (smokers beware!); if on the nose, there could be heart difficulties, perhaps excessive cholesterol; if on the mouth and jaw (often around menstruation many women get an outbreak of pimples on their chin or the surrounding area) the kidneys and reproductive organs may be affected. Excess hair on the chin and/or upper lip, often quite embarrassing for women, also indicates an imbalance within the body. For the removal of excessive or unwanted hair, waxing is the best and safest method. A waxing set costs around $5.00 at chemists and can be used for months with great effect.

Warts and moles in Chinese medicine are a sign of excess. The Chinese believe that moles are found mainly in self-centred people. Excess proteins and animal fats will produce warts. Try some thuja cream externally on warts and garlic tablets internally.

Although to some acupuncture is still not scientifically proven, it has survived over 5000 years in eastern countries. I am a great believer in acupuncture and have seen its results. Several years ago, after having bitten on a large seed in a date, I chipped a tooth and damaged the nerve. Root canal therapy was needed and the dental surgeon – who was open-minded and interested – allowed an acupuncturist to anaesthetise the gums and jaw, so that surgery could be performed. The surgery took 2 hours and with a gold needle in my earlobe and a couple in my feet constantly being stimulated, I felt no pain. I remember the dentist had his needle on standby as he was fully aware of how painful this surgery is. The dental needle was not needed at all and I was only aware of having very cold feet. Afterwards, all I needed was a hot drink.

A Valuable Form of Medicine

I have seen people looking 10 years younger after having facial acupuncture. The needles that are inserted do not hurt. They set up a current of impulses along the meridian triggering a reaction by the central nervous system; this is passed to the lower centres of the brain and then back to the problem area. If no stimulation is needed by the part of the body being treated then it will self-regulate and no danger will be involved.

It is a safe method of treatment and generally for minor problems four to six treatments should suffice. For long-standing problems and those that may be pending, the practitioner will advise approximately how many treatments will be needed. The results often speak for themselves in one or two treatments. A patient's condition should subsequently be assessed every 6 months for proper maintenance and the correction of imbalances.

Acupuncture has had wonderful results in both eastern and western countries, and in cases where a patient's life is endangered by an anaesthetic, it is certainly a wonderful alternative. Skin disorders respond exceptionally well to acupuncture. I have seen acne, psoriasis, eczema, hormonal imbalances and skin discolouration clear up within a few treatments.

9 NATURAL MAKE-UP

Most cosmetics and skin care products on the market are made by companies who test their products on animals. The pain and suffering they endure, just so that people can alter their appearance, does not seem to be justified. Try to buy those products that stress 'No animal has suffered in the manufacture of this product'.

Most cosmetics contain lead or chemicals that over a period of time can set up an irritation. Try your local health shop for the range of natural cosmetics that are available. Some of the colours are unavailable in a natural form, but do shop around.

Making Your Own Cosmetics

Many natural resources for making your own cosmetics are readily available and inexpensive. Cochineal, a food colouring, makes a great pink-red lip gloss if a drop or two is added to your lip gloss. Beetroot juice can also be used as a natural colour. Saffron gives a bright yellow-orange tone when used, but is very expensive and not easy to come by.

The following recipe provides a cheek tint of a very pleasant shade. Beetroot, raw and grated, with the juice expressed into a cup, is left to simmer in a double saucepan. Once the liquid has been reduced to about one-quarter of its original volume, it is ready to be incorporated into some glycerine for the cheek tint. What you will need is as follows:

Beetroot and Glycerine Cheek Tint
　5 ml glycerine
4-6 drops beetroot juice (more, if desired, for a darker colour)
Place in a small glass bottle and shake well.

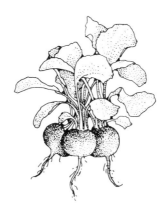

For a lovely natural lip tint or lipstick that may be flavoured with a hint of spearmint, if desired, use the following:

Off-Beet Lipstick
  1 tsp castor oil
  2 tsp beeswax
  4 tsp olive oil
  ½ tsp camphor BP (optional, not readily available)
  ½ tsp beetroot juice
  2 drops spearmint oil or peppermint oil
Melt wax in a double saucepan. Remove from heat and add remaining ingredients. Store in small pots and apply with clean fingertips. Not only is this a great lip colour but it is also wonderful for dry or cracked lips. It can be refrigerated if it melts in the sun.

If your lips are cracked and sore, one of nature's most healing remedies is honey. Honey on the lips, provided you don't lick it off, will create an instant soothing effect and heal quickly. Aloe vera juice applied to the lips will assist in rapid healing also.

A patient of mine has been plagued by a huge varicose ulcer and it initially seemed that nothing short of a skin graft was pending. However, recently a young doctor in America found that honey applied to a wound gave better results than orthodox methods, and that with the same treatment ulcers healed quickly, absorbing moisture and allowing healing to commence. The patient in question is now responding to this honey treatment – chasing away the odd ant, but finding that it really does work. For sores and wounds that need a natural antibiotic (having checked with your doctor first), give the honey treatment a try.

Foundation, Powder and Blusher

Your selection of working materials need not be expensive. Here is a brief list: tissues or Chux cloths, brushes in at least three different sizes, a sponge (to correct make-up lines that come between the face and neck regions), cottonwool and cotton buds, to apply toner and eye shadow.

Your foundation should be as near to the colour of your skin as possible. Before selecting your foundation – and this is a must – use the manufacturer's sample on the smooth part of the inside wrist and walk outside into natural light. You may find that in the store the lighting, as in most buildings, does not show the full spectrum of colours or distorts the appearance of particular shades. Have you ever noticed how your make-up looks fine before you go out and then when you check it somewhere else, it has a different appearance? This is because most ladies' rooms have fluorescent lighting, giving mirror images a rather washed-out appearance.

Once you have selected your foundation, ensure that the test patch has not irritated your skin. If it has, avoid it at all costs, as your skin is telling you that one of the constituents is not right for you. A matching face powder could complement and highlight. Translucent powder is ideal as it does not give your skin that caked-on, overdone look. If applied with a large brush it goes on more evenly and is great as a cover-up for skin pigment variation. The benefit of using a powder is that the foundation will stay on longer, with just occasional touch-ups throughout the day, and it gives a more even tone to the skin.

A blusher is one of the most important highlighters if you are not blessed with lovely rosy cheeks. If you are using a cream foundation and no powder, then a cream blusher works well; if using over powder, then use a powder blusher. Remember to use sparingly to bring out your bone structure and emphasise your features. Nothing looks more false than a blusher that does not suit your colouring. After applying powder and blusher, run your large brush in a downward motion. This helps to flatten those tiny facial hairs that will be standing on end after having applied your foundation in an upward motion. If your skin is fair, avoid the dark burgundy/brown shades and look towards the softer pinks. If your skin is dark olive or brown, then the darker shades will be more applicable for your skin type.

Eye Make-Up

Eye shadows come in such an array of colours that it is hard to know where to begin. Many years ago we were restricted to blues, browns and whites. Today we can mix and match to our heart's desire. Eye shadows come in pencil, cream and powder form. The easiest to apply for some is the powder, others prefer the creams that can have other colours mixed in before applying. With your fine brush, apply a lighter colour around the eyebrow area, with a darker shade on the eyelid. If you are using a pencil or cream, remember that they dry quickly; with your fingertip get the desired shading and then wipe off or smooth the excess with a slightly damp cotton bud.

For an economical eye shadow set, get the primary colours that normally come with a white highlighter and mix up as many different shades as you like – an artist's delight! There are no wrongs or rights in the way people apply make-up. If the end result looks satisfactory to you, then that method is right for you; I have only provided a guideline, which may be varied according to each individual.

Kohl or kajal pencils have been used since early Egyptian times. Those big black eyes we see in many pictures of Egyptian kings, queens and workers indicate the special attention given to their eyes. Kohl pencils are soft and easy to use, and once applied can be smoothed out with the touch of a fingertip. Most pencils these days are waterproof so we rarely have to touch up during the day or evening. Kohl pencil can be used on eyebrows as well as on eyelids. There have been reports that kohl can be carcinogenic due to its charcoal base, but I imagine one would have to use it excessively to find this is so. Perhaps if your eyes are sensitive, or you are prone to allergies, then it should be avoided. Commonsense should always prevail.

Mascara can, like kohl pencil, alter the eyes completely. The colour is entirely up to you but try to use one as close to the colour of your lashes as possible. Mascara is easy to apply. Looking down, apply to top lashes. Looking up, apply to lower lashes. Run brush in a left to right motion if you wish before applying, to separate the hairs. This makes it easier and helps to prevent it from caking on. For those people who wear glasses or contact lenses and find that eye make-up irritates, try applying your powder shadow with a damp brush. This helps to prevent tiny fragments from getting into your eyes and making them watery or irritated. Avoid using pencil on the inner lid area and be sure when buying make-up that it is hypo-allergenic. This will help if any particles do get into the eye.

A good make-up mirror that magnifies will assist those who wear glasses. As each stage of your eye make-up is completed, pop on glasses and check, then continue. Glasses these days look great and have become an important fashion accessory. Perhaps because they are a window over the mirror to the soul, glasses often allow poeple who wear them a better chance to dress up their eyes. The glasses seem to emphasise them!

Skin Care Products

If shopping around for skin care products and vitamins, remember to read labels and ask questions. Do some research yourself to find what suits your skin and why. Expensive creams and lotions are not necessarily the best for your skin. Before outlaying money that may be wasted, try samples, testers and sachets, and within a short time you will know what suits your skin type. Remember also that every 28 days or so new cells are formed, and it could take at least a month before you even begin to see the effect of your perseverance. So be patient and don't be afraid to be a little daring at times: experiment with different combinations until you get the effect you are looking for.

10 SKIN CARE FOR MEN

So many men who come to the clinic ask hesitantly about a skin care regime. It has taken a while for males to be seen in beauty and hair-dressing salons; nowadays we hardly give it a second thought.

Perhaps men need a beauty book more than women, as women can hide a lot of imperfections with make-up, make their eyes look bigger or give themselves high cheek bones with just a little colour. It is acceptable for women, but not for men. Men, unfortunately, have to show all their imperfections. Like women, they are subject to acne, aging, and skin conditions, perhaps more so if they have their hands in grease and grime or are working under heavy stress conditions.

If wives or girlfriends are making up any of the skin care recipes in this book, share some of the ingredients with your menfolk, as most of the recipes will cater for two or more treatments. When I was making up some of the formulas, men were volunteers for each new one tried. Their comments were quite different from those made by women, as they had had little experience with mashed strawberries, essential oils or face masks. The one comment that kept coming through repeatedly was 'That feels great', and many of them have continued to cleanse and tone since then, using oils instead of after-shaves (the latter tend to be quite drying), particularly those which have an oriental fragrance such as sandalwood, myrrh, patchouli and frankincense. A good toner made from lavender water or rosewater with a little witch hazel will close off pores. A little essential oil rubbed on the neck or a drop to anoint between the eyes will give a lasting subtle odour. (Some of the fragrances manufactured for men on a commercial basis are powerful and even nauseating.)

Skin care for men is not costly and a few of the following natural treatments may help.

Hands

If hands are dry and appear dirty, make a mixture of 1 egg yolk and the juice of a medium-sized lemon, and massage well into hands; a soft nail brush will assist. Alternatively, mix together 25 g (1 oz) powdered pumice stone and 25 g (1 oz) powdered Castile soap; apply to wet hands, scrub and wash off.

Lemon juice will whiten hands; it has a tendency to dry skin, so always apply a moisturiser with this treatment. An application of apricot oil and lavender oil will suffice – 50 ml apricot oil, 20 drops lavender oil. The lavender will help to heal rough or peeling skin.

Many men who are in the building trade develop what I call 'brickies' hands': dry, calloused and sore hands. I find the following recipe of great value for this condition, and I dedicate it to all brick-layers, particularly my two brothers-in-law, Steve and David, who come into this category.

Bricklayers Balm

2 tbsp beeswax
40 ml olive oil
28 g pure Castile soap, powdered
20 ml castor oil
7 g powdered pumice stone
5 drops eucalyptus oil
1 tbsp honey
½ cup powdered oatmeal

Place Castile soap powder and beeswax in a double glass saucepan and allow to melt. Add olive oil, castor oil, pumice, eucalyptus oil, oatmeal and honey. Stir all the ingredients together. Pour into a wide necked jar so that your hand can scoop some out. Use often.

Acne and Skin Eruptions

For acne or skin eruptions on the back, chest and face, cleanse off dead skin with a body brush and apply the following mixture:

½ cup powdered oatmeal
¼ cup fuller's earth
4 drops benzoin
pinch cinnamon

Mix all the ingredients together with enough water to form the consistency of runny porridge. Get a friend to apply to affected areas, leave on for 15 minutes or until dry. Shower off. This will draw and exfoliate dead tissue.

The above should be done at least once a week or until skin shows an improvement. Tea-tree oil diluted in some castor oil (around 4 drops tea-tree oil to 25 ml castor oil) can be applied to affected areas with a cotton bud or cottonwool after the mask.

Feet

For tinea or athlete's foot, massage a few drops of lavender oil onto affected areas daily; this acts as a natural antibiotic. Tea-tree oil added also helps with its antifungal properties. Try a combination of both diluted in olive oil, 25 ml to 4 drops of tea-tree oil.

For Body Odours

If you happen to suffer from strong body odour and perspiration, add 1 drop of lavender oil under each arm. This will last for a few hours. A drop of lavender or patchouli oil on the soles of the feet is an ideal way to keep odour away.

Cleansing Skin

To draw blackheads and grime, make the following solution and apply twice daily:

1 tsp Epsom salts (dissolved in 10 ml boiled water)
6 drops benzoin
10 ml witch hazel
Mix all the ingredients together and with a cotton ball, dab and compress the cottonwool on affected area for 2 to 3 minutes.

A good face mask once every 1 or 2 weeks will remove dead tissue, leaving the face glowing as stimulation of circulation is evident from the first treatment:
1 eggwhite
5 drops aloe vera juice (optional)
1 tsp honey
Mix all the ingredients together and apply in upward strokes, avoiding the eye and upper lip area. Do not forget the neck and chin area. Lean head back so that honey does not run down face. Leave on for 15 to 20 minutes or until dry. Use this time to relax; close eyes and switch off from all thoughts. Rinse off with warm water. Tone with a little witch hazel and apply a moisturiser. This feels fantastic and makes the skin look and feel alive.

If your skin is dry, or has any open wound or sore, avoid using this recipe as it could burn or sting. Always try a patch test if your skin is sensitive; the back of the wrist is ideal.

Applying face packs, aromatherapy and reflexology massage is not only therapeutic but fun if your mate joins in and you make it a team effort.

Moisturising and Toning Skin

For a really good moisturising cream, the following is easy and effective:

2 tsp beeswax
2 tsp lanolin
2 tsp castor oil
pinch borax
1 tsp wheatgerm oil
1 drop lavender oil

In a double saucepan combine beeswax, lanolin and castor oil and stir until melted. In 2 teaspoons warm water, add borax and allow to cool. When both mixtures have cooled add wheatgerm oil and lavender oil to the beeswax mixture, then mix all the ingredients together. Store in an airtight jar. To make a larger quantity, double the mixture. This oil is great to apply after a day in the sun or surf. If applied prior to going into the sun, then skin will still burn – so be careful. As a night cream, it is invaluable.

For a quick, revitalising bath, add 4 tablespoons baking soda to the water and 2 drops of rosemary oil. It is a great 'pick-me-up'. For a quick facial tone-up, try this:

1 egg
½ avocado
1 tsp mayonnaise

Place all the ingredients into a blender and mix thoroughly. Apply to neck and face. Leave on for 15 minutes, then rinse off. The addition of a teaspoon of honey makes it a moisturiser as well. This should leave your skin feeling alive and silky soft. It will not keep, so share it with a friend if you don't use it all.

Treating Burns

If you happen to burn your skin apply lavender oil instantly to the affected area. Its natural antibiotic properties prevent infection and the healing property of lavender soothes the burning and promotes rapid healing. By coincidence, as I was writing this section my next door neighbour's son and his friend were working on a car motor when it caught fire. The friend received burns on his arm. I applied lavender oil instantly and followed this by an ice-pack. The benefits were immediately obvious. Aloe vera juice applied to burns will also bring relief.

Infected Hair Follicles

Infected hair follicles can lead to red, raised and very sore skin infections. Using a very warm flannel that has been soaked in boiled water, add 1 drop of eucalyptus oil to the water and leave flannel on the area for a few seconds. Repeating the action several times will help to draw impurities. With tweezers (boiled for 5 minutes in water and allowed to cool), pull hair out and apply further hot flannels and eucalyptus oil. With a clean cotton ball, dab witch hazel onto area to help close off open pores. Lavender oil will assist in keeping away further infection and assist with rapid healing. Apply this daily.

After the skin has healed, follow the above recipe with a mixture of 1 cup oatmeal and 2 tablespoons ground almonds, reduced to a fine powder in a blender or mortar and pestle and made into a paste by adding water. This is great for removing dead skin, dirt and grime.

If you feel you need a little assistance to get started with these treatments, get your girlfriend, mother or wife to help – the treatments are really very straightforward and well worth trying!

11 HAIR CARE FOR WOMEN AND MEN

Hair consists of around 97 per cent protein, the remaining 3 per cent being moisture. Hair-roots lie below the surface of the skin in the small sac-shaped glands known as follicles. The function of each follicle is to produce keratin, a protein substance. An oil gland supplies a coating to each strand of hair to protect moisture in that strand. If we are healthy inwardly then this function will be carried out properly. If we become sick, our glands congested or hormones erratic, then the hair will suffer. Sometimes the hair just looks dull and lacking lustre, at other times it may fall out in clumps (particularly after glandular fever or chemotherapy). This does not mean it will not grow back, but the success rate will depend on the internal structure; after all, hair, like nails, is a 'dead' substance. It is the follicle that has 'life' and this feeds via the papilla, which receives nourishment via the bloodstream. If we are deficient in zinc, calcium or B group vitamins, then often these deficiencies will create hair loss or dull hair.

Perming, tinting and blow-drying put a lot of stress onto normally healthy hair and over a period of time will create brittle hair or hair loss. Dyes and colour changes can strip the protective coating from hair, making it break or split. However, if these things are done in moderation very little damage will occur. It is normal to lose between 100 to 200 hairs daily, as we have an average of 100 000 hairs on our head. One of the safest colourings to use, in terms of being non-toxic, is henna powder. Henna, once you experiment with it, can produce some of the loveliest colours I have ever seen, from the blue-black shades to the rich copper and mahogany tones.

The colour of henna, which is a reddy-brown mixture, can be darkened or lightened depending on what it is mixed with. Added to 1 cup of henna powder, 2 teaspoons of coffee will give it a brown tone; the more coffee, the darker the hair will become. To lighten henna, the juice of a lemon and an egg should be added. A teaspoon of vinegar will assist in releasing the colour of henna. Henna will create a deeper shade if left on for up to 3 hours. Once the mixture has been made into a paste, simply by adding water, the hair is then sectioned off and wrapped in plastic food wrap to hold the henna on the hair and avoid staining. Hands and nails should be protected as the dye will colour the skin. For that rich, red tone, add a pinch of saffron to the powder before applying. Clean hair will always take colour best, so be quite sure than you shampoo well before applying the henna.

The pH balance of the hair should be approximately 5.5. If we subject it to harsh chemicals or detergents that are too alkaline we cause a change in the acid mantle or protective covering. Swimming pools with chlorine often leave our hair 'green' or brittle and this is because it allows the follicle to open up and the shaft of hair swells. If your shampoo is around the same pH balance as your hair – preferably slightly acidic – then disruption that leads to dull hair or hair loss will be prevented. Medications, antibiotics and the like will affect the condition of the hair; these are internal stress-related problems which show quickly on the outside. The contraceptive pill has been known to cause hair problems and this is due to the hormonal changes that greatly influence the state of our hair. Always take B group vitamins while taking the contraceptive pill.

Herbal Mixtures for the Hair

Home hair remedies that will show results very quickly can be made from rosemary, yarrow, horsetail, chamomile, nettle or sage. After collecting your herbs, bruise and pour boiling water over them; leave this to steep for a couple of hours and then strain and use the water as a final rinse after shampooing. Alternatively, saturate the hair, wrap plastic food wrap around the head and leave for 20 minutes; towel dry hair and brush. Sage will darken grey hair. Apply daily and leave on for 15 minutes.

To keep the hair looking healthy and to prevent loss of hair, pick a handful of sage and rosemary leaves. Bruise them and pour over 2 cups of boiling water. Allow to steep for an hour. Strain and massage into scalp. This mixture will keep refrigerated for several days.

A mixture of crushed rosemary and lavender makes a delightful hair rinse and if you have a good quality hair shampoo, it can be incorporated also into the cleansing, as well as into the rinsing of the hair. The combination of rosemary and lavender creates a wonderful, refreshing smell that seems to linger on the hair, and people often comment that my hair smells nice after I have used this mixture.

A combination of chamomile flowers, lavender and nettle will suit the fair-haired person. Pick a cup of each and bruise them, or use your mortar and pestle to break them up. Pour 3 cups boiling water over bruised herbs and steep for 2 hours. After washing hair, rinse with the strained water. If you sit in the sun while brushing hair it will highlight the natural fairness and bring out the most beautiful sheen.

Remember that too much sun will damage and dry the hair, causing it to lose its lustre.

Try to avoid using plastic brushes and combs as these tend to split hair endings. A good bristle brush and tortoise shell comb will benefit the hair and an old silk scarf or stocking placed over the bristles will bring the sheen out on dull hair.

Check with your hairdresser to find out what condition your hair is in, if you are not sure. If you have an oily scalp but the ends of the hair are dry, then maybe the use of a dry shampoo would assist.

Orris root powder (which is used in potpourri) or arrowroot powder make an excellent dry shampoo. Cover your brush with a silk scarf and sprinkle about ¼ to ½ teaspoon orris root powder or arrowroot on the brush. Brush your hair for about 5 minutes, or until all the powder has been absorbed by the oil in the hair. This is great when you don't have enough time to wash or maintain your hair properly, or if you happen to be travelling or in hospital. Lemon juice massaged into the scalp will prevent an oily scalp. Brushing the hair with a good brush will generally help distribute the oil to the ends that become dry and brittle.

Your hair is your 'crowning glory' and although to a large extent its appearance reflects your internal state of health, we can do a great deal externally to improve its appearance.

More money is spent on hair styling and hair care today than the barber of yesteryear could ever have imagined possible. Today we think nothing of seeing men having their hair permed or tinted at the hairdressers. Hair care (as well as skin care and clothing) is often just as important to men as it is to women. The remedies included in this chapter, therefore, are for men as well as for women.

Oils for the Hair

People often ask, 'How will this particular oil help my hair or skin?' By using essential oils and mixing them with a pure vegetable oil that dilutes and allows easy spreading, the essential oil is absorbed through the bloodstream and the lymphatic system. Always be sure that the oils you are using are pure and not of a synthetic origin, as synthetic oils are sometimes labelled essential oils. There are several reputable firms which supply pure oils and prices vary according to demand and availability.

Always use a base made from vegetable oil, not mineral oil as these inhibit the working of essential oils. Oils that are used to treat oily skin and imbalances work quickly and effectively.

If your hair is very oily the following recipe will help:

50 ml sesame oil
15 drops bergamot oil
15 drops lavender oil
10 drops rosemary oil
5 drops pine oil
Combine the oils. Section the hair into easy working parts. With cottonwool, begin at the root end and continue until all hair has been saturated. I warm the oil prior to application as it seems to spread more easily. Wrap plastic food wrap around head or use a plastic shower cap to contain the oil. Wrap a towel over the plastic and leave on for 1 to 2 hours. When ready, apply shampoo and rinse off. If this is repeated weekly it will assist in balancing the oil secretions.

For dry hair, apply the following using the above method:

50 ml sesame oil as a base
20 drops rosewood oil
20 drops lavender oil
5 drops patchouli oil
2 vitamin E capsules

For Permed or Bleached Hair

50 ml sesame oil as a base
10 drops geranium oil
10 drops sandalwood oil
20 drops rosewood oil
5 drops lavender oil
1 vitamin E capsule (oil)
1 vitamin A capsule (oil)
Apply as for oily hair.

Rosemary has been a hair remedy for centuries. Oil of rosemary massaged a few drops at a time will leave hair shining and healthy. For a rosemary protein conditioner take:

1 egg yolk
½ cup warm apricot kernel oil
4 drops rosemary oil
2 tsp olive oil
Mix together, massage into hair and leave on for 15 to 20 minutes. Wrap a towel around the hair to avoid drips and shampoo with a good pH balanced shampoo.

A very good protein conditioner is the yolk of an egg beaten with ½ cup castor oil. Massage the mixture into the scalp, leave for 15 minutes, wash off and rinse with rosemary water. If this is done weekly the condition of the hair will improve greatly. I have seen this treatment work on the most stubborn cases of scale and dandruff. Rosemary oil assists circulation and may also be used to treat a persistant headache; try rubbing a few drops into the forehead or any other painful area. This oil has been used throughout the ages, surviving the test of time as a remedy for the hair and head. Amulets used to be worn with dried rosemary to drive away pains in the head.

For Head Lice, apply the following remedy:

4 drops sassafras oil
2 drops pennyroyal oil
5 ml sesame oil
Mix all the ingredients together and warm oil. Section hair, apply and then comb through with a fine comb. Leave on overnight and once again comb through with a fine comb. Head lice should be dead and eggs will come out easily. Repeat weekly for 2 weeks if necessary; however, the first application is generally all that is needed. Remember orris root powder sprinkled onto hair will absorb grease and is ideal as a dry shampoo.

Many people who have trees, flowers and herbs growing at home may not be aware of the qualities and potential uses of some of their plants.

If you are lucky enough to have a walnut tree growing in your garden, or you know someone who does, pick a handful of these leaves, and a cup of ivy leaves, pound them together with 25 ml of castor oil or olive oil, then strain. Repeat these actions until you have around ½ cup of green oil. Massage through hair. The left-over portion may be refrigerated. The oil you use on your hair may be warmed before mixing it with the walnut and ivy leaves. It may also be warmed after you have mixed it with the leaves. This treatment is excellent for itchy scalp, dandruff and as a protein booster treatment. It brings warm brown tones to the hair.

The eucalyptus (gum) tree yields an invaluable oil that is a powerful antiseptic. Try the following remedy for dandruff; it can also be used for chapped hands, swollen glands, stiffness in muscles and joints, and problem skin.

Dandruff Remover
25 ml castor oil
12 drops eucalyptus oil
5 drops oil of wintergreen
Mix the three oils together, warm and apply to hair. (For sore joints, apply a poultice using a flannel soaked in warm water over the area you have oiled. Place a hot water bottle over the flannel and leave until the heat has gone from the bottle. Repeat daily.)

A few drops of olive oil massaged into the scalp will assist in removing dandruff and cradle cap on small babies.

Bay rum, popular in grandmother's day, has just as many followers today, and is combined with three oils in the following hair tonic:

Bay Rum Hair Tonic
224 ml (8 fl oz) pure alcohol
28 ml Jamaican rum
40 drops oil of bay
1 drop oil of mace
20 drops oil of orange
water to make up to 452 ml (16 fl oz)
Mix all the ingredients together, shaking occasionally, and leave to stand for 3 weeks. Filter the contents through magnesia and you have the finished product. An alternative to the above is:

224 ml (8 fl oz) pure alcohol
10 ml oil of bay
1 drop oil of cloves
20 drops (or 20 grains mace) oil of mace
water warmed to approx. 25°C (80°F), enough to make 336 ml
Dissolve the oils in the alcohol and leave to stand for 3 days. (Place mace in whole and then filter after 3 days.) Filter through muslin and add the water. Leave to stand again, with occasional agitation, for several days, then filter through magnesia.

12 PLANTS AND THEIR USES – A DIRECTORY

Almond (*Amygdalus dulcis*)   The kernel of the almond is the medicinal part of the plant. Almond oil is widely used in cosmetics. Almond milk is formed by pounding the almonds in water – an enjoyable drink as well as being good for the skin.

Aloe (*Aloe vera*)   The juice from the leaves of this plant is widely used for skin irritations, sunburn and acne. It has a soothing and emollient effect on the skin. This plant is easy to look after and one well worth having in your garden.

Anise (*Pimpinella anisum*)   The fruit of this plant's seed is used. It has a soothing effect on the stomach and the seeds may be chewed after a meal of fish or lamb. After making a tea and steeping for an hour, dab onto skin or acne. A mixture of anise, pennyroyal and sassafras oil is a great deterrent for insects and cockroaches.

Arnica (*Arnica montana*)   The flowers of the arnica plant are used widely in skin toners and for healing wounds. A poultice may be made with the flowers after steeping. Arnica water has a soothing effect when used as a lip balm, or after a cold when the nose is irritated, as it works quickly. Do not take internally as it is a powerful poison if overdosed. Internal administration must be supervised by a homeopath.

Arrowroot (*Maranta arundinaceae*)   The rhizomes of the arrowroot are pounded in a mortar, washed and strained until starch is produced. This has many culinary uses. It makes excellent powders and deodorants with the addition of essential oils and orris root powder.

Avens water (*Geum rivale*)   The root of this plant has a strong astringent action. Avens water can be mixed with witch hazel for a good toner. It has a purple colour when in flower.

Balm (*Melissa officinalis*)   Commonly known as sweet balm or lemon balm, this herb makes a wonderful tea that helps catarrh and high fever. The essential balsam oil is used in potpourri and perfumes. Much used in aromatherapy for allergies and asthma and great for menstrual problems.

Balm or Balsam of Giliad (*Commiphora opobalsamum*)   A sweet smelling oil is produced from the liquid resin of the plant. It can be dissolved in alcohol and used in ointments for bruising and swelling.

Balsam of Peru (*Myroxylon pereirae*)   This oily liquid from the plant can be used for skin disorders, including eczema or itching. It can be applied directly to the skin or mixed in a good base cream for troubled skin. It makes the most beautiful, creamy, sweet-smelling soap.

Basil, sweet (*Ocymum basilium*)   This is one of the plants used to draw poison from the skin. It is widely used as a poultice after wasp or bee stings. It also benefits those underlying pimples and brings them quickly to a head. The whole herb is used; it has a pleasant smell and is recommended for use in potpourris. A great tonic for congested skin.

Beetroot (*Beta chenopodiaceae*)   The root of this plant is most commonly used, but the leaves can also be used. Beetroot is well known as a cleanser of the body, particularly the liver and spleen. It has been used to provide natural dyes for lipstick and rouge. Rinsing the hair in beetroot juice will assist with itchy scalp and dandruff. Beetroot is an energy-giver for the body. Grate a beetroot and have it raw in a salad or mix with onion and carrot; it tastes great.

Benzoin (*Styrax benzoin*)   Incisions are made in the stem of the tree to allow the liquid benzoin to seep through the incision and harden. It is then collected for preparations such as compound benzoin, the tincture being used for bronchial ailments and inhalants. It is used for many skin products, and is found to be invaluable for boils, abscesses and pimples. Blackheads respond well to benzoin tincture, as does eczema, dermatitis, itching or redness.

Bergamot (*Monarda didyma*)   Bergamot leaves, fruit and flowers are used in sachets and potpourris. The herb yields a beautiful sweet perfume and is used in many fragrances for soaps and perfumes. A tea, called Oswego tea, is made from the fresh young leaves. It appears to be calming for the system. It is effective against tuberculosis bacilli and infections, and is used to flavour Earl Grey tea. Its name derives from the citrus bergamia, the rind of the fruit being used.

Birch (*Betula alba*)   When the twigs of this tree are crushed or bruised, the smell of oil of wintergreen may come to mind. Birch oil is marketed on a commercial basis as oil of wintergreen. It brings relief to sore muscles and joints and has astringent and antiseptic qualities. It is also a good insect repellent and can be mixed with olive oil and massaged over the body to relieve aches and pains.

Cajuput (*Melaleuca leucadendron*)   The oil is distilled from the leaves of the plant and is widely used throughout the East for psoriasis, eczema, rheumatic pain and itchy skin. It has strong antiseptic qualities.

Castor oil plant (*Ricinus communis*)   The seeds of the castor oil plant are 'cold pressed' in hydraulic presses to obtain the oil. Castor oil is an invaluable item to have on hand to use as a castor-oil pack for the skin, for sore and aching muscles, and to protein the hair with the addition of essential oils. The list of uses for this incredible oil is endless. (The seeds, if eaten, are poisonous, however.)

Celandine (*Chelidonium majus*)   When the stem and leaves of this herb are broken away, a juice flows freely. This juice can be applied to a vitamin E base cream and rubbed into irritated skin and eczema. The orange-coloured juice can stain the skin, so use with caution.

Chamomile (*Anthemis nobilis*)   The dried flowers and leaves of this herb are used for many purposes: as a calming tea for children, to make the hair glow and as a lotion for pain in the neuralgic nerve and tooth and ear aches. It makes a lovely base for a herbal sleep pillow. The oil is good for the liver. It is also an anti-allergic remedy for skin allergies.

Cinnamon (*Cinnamomum zeylanicum*)   The inner bark of this small tree's twigs is distilled to yield small amounts of cinnamon oil. The spice of the plant was formerly used to trade and bargain with, and was once more valuable than gold. The powder can be mixed into scrubs and sachets. The oil may be added to a little almond oil and gently massaged over the face. It has a relaxing quality when inhaled.

Clary Sage (*Salvia sclarea*)   This plant is useful in an oil form for potpourris and sachets. It is used as a fixative and in aromatherapy for menstrual problems and childbirth. It has anti-inflammatory properties for the skin, particularly dry skin.

Cucumber (*Cucumis sativa*)   The whole fruit is used. Cut into slices and placed on the skin, it has soothing and healing qualities. When made into a lotion with a little lemon juice, it becomes a toner and astringent.

Echinacea (*Echinacea augustifolia*)   The root and rhizome are used. It has long had the reputation of being a cleanser and purifier of the system. It is used for skin disorders and eczema. As a tea, it improves digestion.

Elder (*Sambucus nigra*)   The bark, leaves, flowers and berries are used for skin disorders. Elder flower water can be used as a face wash, left on the skin to dry, then rinsed off. As a compress, soak a flannel in the flower water. It has been used for every imaginable ailment, including headache, throughout recorded history. Elder leaves are used in ointments for bruises, sprains, rheumatism and sore joints.

Elecampane (*Inula helenium*)   The root is used for many skin washes and skin disorders. Internally it is used as a purifier and for bronchial disorders. It will repel insects if burnt. In America, it is used externally for sciatica and neuralgia.

Eucalyptus (*Eucalyptus globulus*)   The oil of the leaves is used. The distilled oil is antiseptic and aromatic. It is used externally and internally. Externally applied to infections, ulcers and pimples, it has strong healing qualities. A mixture of 10 ml castor oil, 2 drops oil of wintergreen and 2 drops eucalyptus oil, rubbed into muscular aches and pains, brings great relief. Eucalyptus oil is a wonderful inhaler and eases congestion in nasal passages. It makes a refreshing gargle and soothes irritated throats. It reduces body heat by cooling the system, and is antiseptic and diuretic in its properties.

Fennel (*Foeniculum vulgare*)   This plant is more than just a culinary delight. The seeds, leaves and roots are used. Fennel is used to make fragrances for many soaps or perfumes. It makes a pleasant tea and has diuretic properties. Fennel seeds chewed after a fatty meal will soothe and help with digestion. Fennel aids weight loss if you are dieting. It increases milk production if you are nursing a baby.

Frankincense (*Boswellia thurifera*)   This is the aromatic gum resin yielded by various trees, in particular Egyptian women make 'kohl' for the eyes out of burnt or charred frankincense. The oil is an essential part of many oriental perfumes, soaps and cosmetics. It has held significant religious attributes throughout history. To the present day, it is burnt as incense in many churches. It has rejuvenating qualities and is a great addition to a moisturiser or mask.

Galbanum (*Ferula galbaniflua*)   The gum resin yields a thick oil that has soothing and anti-inflammatory properties.

Garlic (*Allium sativum*)   The bulb is the part used internally and externally. Cloves of garlic form the bulb. Garlic oil is rich in sulphur and acts as a purifier, and conditioner for troubled skin. The raw juice dabbed onto acne and wounds promotes rapid healing.

Geranium (*Pelargonium crispum*)   The oil of this plant is invaluable for perfumes and soaps. It gives body to sachets and potpourris. The leaves can be made into tea or used as a face wash and toner. It is used extensively for wounds and sores, eczema and dry skin, shingles and inflamed skin.

Golden seal (*Hydrastis canadensis*)   Belonging to the buttercup family, golden seal is used for ulcers and wounds, to promote rapid healing. It works on the mucous membrane and powdered golden seal has been used for centuries as a snuff.

Henna (*Lawsonia inermis*) The fruit, flowers and leaves, powdered, are all used in various ways. The powdered leaves make a conditioner and dye for the hair and nails. The flowers are sweet smelling and ideal for herbal sachets. The fruit in days gone by was considered a remedy for women who suffered from miscarriage.

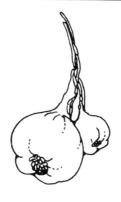

Honeysuckle (*Lonicera caprifolium*)   The honeysuckle produces a sweet perfume used in cosmetics, perfumes and potpourri. It has been much used for ailments of the bronchial system and it is relaxing when inhaled. The leaves, flowers and seeds are used internally and externally.

Hops (*Humulus lupulus*)   The flowers, when dried and placed in a herbal pillow, promote sleep. (Lavender dried and added to the pillow gives it a more pleasing odour.) Hops have a calming effect on the system when made into herb beer.

Horseradish (*Cochlearia armoracia*)   The root of the plant is frequently used in the kitchen to make horseradish sauce. Taken internally it assists in clearing the sinus passages and eliminating mucus. It is a stimulant for the digestive system. It can be applied as a poultice to reduce swellings.

Ivy (*Hedera helix*)   The leaves make an excellent astringent and work well as ivy soap for cellulite. Made as a poultice it has soothing qualities and is said to be a deterrent for wrinkles.

Jasmine (*Jasminum odoratissimum*)   The flowers make a lovely tea well known in China. There are many varieties of jasmine. The flower is effectively used for sachets, aromatherapy and potpourri. It gives a lingering fragrance to soap and powder.

Laurel, Bay (*Laurus nobilis*)   The leaves are infused to make a calming tea. The oil is massaged into sprains and strains.

Lavender (*Lavandula officinalis*)   The leaves and flowers are mainly used for their purifying and antiseptic properties. Lavender oil can be applied directly to the skin; a drop rubbed under the arm or added to arrowroot makes a deodorant. It is said that an amulet worn around the neck, with lavender and rosemary, relieves headache. In days of old, lavender was used to purify the streets. Lavender strengthens the blood. Smelling lavender will restore health when feeling faint. Good for leg ulcers and wounds.

Lemon (*Citrus limonum*)   The juice, rind and oil are used for perfume and medicine. Lemon juice whitens the skin and makes a good toner for oily skin. The dried leaves and flowers are used mainly in the production of perfume and medicine. Lemon juice, taken in warm water each morning, assists cleansing processes. Add a little ginger and honey and use as a tonic for sore throats or irritating coughs and colds. Dried lemon powder assists the healing of wounds and ulcers.

Mace (*Myristica fragrans*)   This is the dried outer covering of nutmeg. The oil is used in perfume and potpourri. It is soothing for the stomach, aids digestion and is helpful for arthritis when used as a massage.

Marigold (*Calendula officinalis*)   The flowers and leaves are used. Marigold flowers can be applied directly to a bite or sting, and they add a lovely colour to potpourri. Calendula cream is a great aid for eczema and irritated skin. Marigolds are invaluable when made into a hair wash for dandruff and itchy scalp. Marigold juice applied to warts will help remove them.

Marjoram, sweet (*Origanum marjorana*)   This herb is used both internally and externally. It is a culinary delight and steeped in vinegar and garlic makes a lovely salad dressing. It helps soothe the nervous system and can be rubbed onto the sinus region for conges-tion and headache. If you are inclined to 'sigh' constantly, it relieves anxiety of the heart, particularly if one is suffering from grief.

Melissa *See* **Balm**

Myrrh (*Commiphora myrrha*)   This is an aromatic gum resin of the tree. It is obtained by making incisions in the tree or from natural cracks and fissures. From a thick pale yellow oil it hardens to a reddish brown colour. It has been used for thousands of years in temples and religious institutions, in anointing oils, perfumes and ointments. It has anti-inflammatory properties. Healing wounds and ulcers and ulcerated throats will benefit greatly. Myrrh oil added to a moisturiser or vegetable oil will cleanse and tighten the skin. Myrrh oil helps circu-lation and is therefore valuable when used as a massage oil.

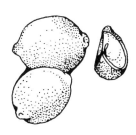

Nettle (*Urtica urens*) The leaves, roots and seeds of the plant are used. It is widely used in tincture and powder form for homeopathic and herbal medicine. It is often mixed in animal food, particularly for horses, to give the coat a glowing healthy appearance. Nettle shampoo or nettle water is good for psoriasis on the scalp or dandruff. Nettle juice may be used directly on the scalp as a tonic and hair restorer. The juice of the roots or leaves mixed with a little honey helps relieve congestion of the bronchial system. Nettle has been used widely for asthma.

Nutmeg (*Myristica fragrans*) The dried kernel of the seed produces the powder which can be pressed and heated to produce 'oil of mace'. Distillation of nutmeg produces the volatile superior oil. It has a calming effect on the gastrointestinal system and is widely used in face masks and medicine. Nutmeg mixed with a little vegetable oil or butter is good for rheumatic pain and haemorrhoids.

Olive (*Olea europaea*) One could write a book on the uses of this ancient tree. The leaves and bark are used as well as the oil of the fruit. If rosemary, fennel or garlic is steeped in olive oil it becomes far more palatable. Olive oil has long been used internally for gall stones and constipation. It helps to disperse acid and cleans the system. Externally it relieves inflammation, bites and stings. Mixed with a little alcohol it makes a hair restorer and an astringent for dry or oily skin. Olive oil helps to detoxify poison from the system and it is widely used for lotions and ointments. Castile soap is generally made from pure olive oil. The Bible mentions the olive tree as a symbol of peace.

Orange, sweet (*Citrus aurantium*), **Bitter orange** (*Citrus vulgaris*) The fruit, flowers and peel are used. The volatile oil produced from the peel of the bitter orange peel is known as Oil of Bigarade; that from the sweet orange is known as Oil of Portugal. The flowers of the bitter orange tree supply the essence for Neroli oil, a non-irritating oil which tones and purifies the skin. This oil also assists in exfoliating the skin and helps greatly on a cellular level. It is used widely in perfume, soap and aromatherapy and has strong calming properties. A bath with a few drops of Neroli oil is great for insomnia. Petigrain Oil is obtained from the leaves of the bitter orange.

Parsley (*Petroselinum crispum*) The whole herb is used in both culinary and medicinal applications. Parsley tea works on the kidney and bladder. It is useful for kidney stones and fluid retention. Parsley contains vitamin C and iron and should be incorporated into the daily diet for general health.

Patchouli (*Pogostemon patchouly*)   The leaves are distilled to produce this heavily scented oriental fragrance. The Arabs employ it to dispel fleas and lice from bedding. It is used in making fragrances for perfumes, soaps and cosmetics. It is also an ingredient in incense for religious ceremonies and is said to have a stimulating effect on the sexual instinct, although this varies with each individual. It is used for redness of the skin, cracking and dry skin and to stimulate sluggishness of the brain.

Pawpaw (*Carica papaya*)   Seeds, leaves, fruit and juice are all used internally and externally. The juice of the pawpaw can be applied directly to the face or the ripe fruit, mashed with a little added honey and rose oil, and makes a wonderful mask. The fresh leaves can be made into a poultice to dress wounds and slow-to-heal sores and ulcers. The juice of the fruit may be an aid to digestive problems as it helps to alkalise the system.

Pennyroyal (*Mentha pulegium*)   This herb has a very strong mint odour. It can be used in cooking and helps to ease earache and tinnitus. Taken internally as a tea it brings on delayed menstruation. Externally it relieves burning and itching skin. A little pennyroyal and sassafras oil will rid your pet of fleas. When used with a vegetable oil the body may be rubbed with pennyroyal oil to dispel fleas, ticks and other biting insects. The whole herb is used.

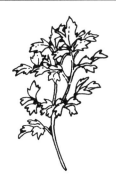

Pepper(*Piper nigrum*)   The peppercorns or fruit of the tree are used. Pepper is used for congestive conditions; it is employed in some countries as a snuff for faintness and nose bleeds, and is antitoxic in some cases of food poisoning. Pepper helps to stimulate the spleen and circulation. It is well worth trying for arthritic pain, as a poultice or massage oil.

Peppermint (*Mentha piperita*)   This herb is used for many flavourings in sweets, toothpaste, teas and medicine. It is one of the most important therapeutic oils. If you suffer from any of the following, then it will assist you: sinusitis, toothache, bad breath, vertigo, migraine, flatulence, hysteria, colic or cough, dry red irritated skin or ringworm. Dilute 1 part peppermint in 99 parts of vegetable oil, glycerine or castor oil, and massage into skin. Peppermint tea, taken internally two or three times daily, cleanses and sweetens stagnation within.

Pine (*various species*)   Pine trees are tapped to produce a resin which is then distilled into oil of turpentine. This oil is used extensively in ointments and liniments for rheumatic pain, muscular aches and sprains and as an antiseptic. The larch pine (*Pinus larix*) is the most commonly used for skin disorders, psoriasis and eczema.

Pipsissewa (*Chimaphila umbellata*)   The dried leaves steeped in boiled water can be applied to skin irritations and disorders and is said to be highly effective. It is used internally in medicine for cysts and kidney complaints.

Potato (*Solanum tuberosum*)   The tubers are the only part of the plant used; the stem, leaves and berries are narcotic and poisonous. The potato consists mainly of starch but it is not always used as an edible commodity. Potato juice has long been used in the treatment of gout and rheumatic pain; it may be added to a little oil and massaged into affected areas of pain. Strains and bruises also respond very well to this treatment. Mashed potato can be made into a poultice for scalds and burns.

Pumpkin seed (*Cucurbita pepo*)   Dried pumpkin seeds are an excellent wormer for the body and can be safely given to animals and children. It is a wonderful regulator for congestion of the male prostate. Try frying pumpkin seeds in a little vegetable oil and packing them in school lunches. They taste a little like roasted almonds. Toss some into your salad for a delicious nutty taste.

Ragweed (*Ambrosa trifida*)   The pollen of the plant is used extensively in homeopathic medicine for hayfever. The plant is astringent and antiseptic. It can be used as a gargle and mouth wash for sore throats and ulcers.

Rose: Cabbage rose (*Rosa centifolia*); Damask rose (*Rosa damascena*); Red rose (*Rosa gallica*)   The rose is not only beautiful to look at, but also has many qualities that are not so well known. Roses are a symbol of love and beauty. Medicinally they are a tonic, anti-depressant, astringent, laxative and aphrodisiac. In olden days roses were used to cleanse, perfume and help the head after consuming too much alcohol. The Damask rose from Bulgaria is the most commonly used for rose oil, or Otto of Rose, and is one of the finest (and most expensive) around. Rosewater and rose oil will assist in menstrual problems for women and infertility in males. Clinical tests in the USSR have shown it to have very high antiseptic qualities, and very little toxicity. It helps to strengthen the capillaries and improve digestion. The leaves of the plant are also used and the tree-oil has great benefits for the mature skin or for inflammation and red, angry-looking pimples. Rose petals can be added to a salad, eaten in a sandwich, made into jam or added to a sachet or potpourri to make it a little more special.

Rosemary (*Rosmarinus officinalis*)   The herb and root are both used internally and externally. It is analgesic, antiseptic, antispasmodic, astringent, calming, digestive, diuretic, stimulating and sudorific. Its name comes from the Latin *ros marinus*, meaning 'sea dew'. Rosemary helps to normalise high cholesterol and is a wonderful tonic for the liver and blood. Applied externally it is a good remedy for muscular weakness and rheumatic pain.

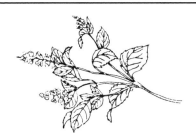

Safflower (*Carthamus tinctorius*)   The seeds of the flower produce an oil that is used for cooking. Its chief constituent is the dye that it produces: both yellow and red. Saffron colouring is often mixed with orris powder to produce red rouge. A flower water to soothe skin irritations may be used internally or dabbed on externally. The saffron produced by the safflower is inferior to that of the saffron plant (*Crocus sativus*).

St John's wort (*Hypericum perforatum*)   An oil made from the flowers of this herb infused in olive oil has been used for many eruptive skin conditions. A poultice made from the herb tops and flowers and applied to swelling will help to disperse it. The oil massaged into breasts will help dry, cracking nipples. Add a drop of rose oil for an extra boost.

Sandalwood (*Santalum album*)   The wood and oil are the parts used from this beautiful tree. After the tree has been dug up and its branches removed, it is graded and produced commercially. The oil is widely used for perfumes, soaps, incense and aromatherapy. Internally it is used, 1 drop on a little brown sugar, for bronchial disorders. It is a great tonic when the oil (Mysore) is applied to dry skin. It also has calming qualities for the nervous system. The Australian sandalwood (*Santalum spicatum*), produces an oil which is also used medicinally; although inferior to the Mysore oil, it is closer to the latter than is the oil produced by the West Indian sandalwood (*Schimmelia olerfera*).

Sassafras (*Sassafras officinale*)   The root bark produces a volatile oil which is used for rheumatism, skin disease and as an insect repellent. It is used in miniscule doses due to its strength and should be prescribed for internal use by your practitioner.

Sedge, sweet (*Acorus calamus*)   The root is the part used. It is an aquatic-looking plant and has long been called by its specific name, calamus. The root stock or rhizome is used for medicinal purposes. The oil is obtained by steam distillation and is much used in perfumery for its aromatic essence. It assists in clearing and head when used as an inhalation, taken internally it relieves flatulence, and it is also used as antiseptic. It has been employed in tooth powders and snuff, and has soothing qualities for the nervous system.

Self-heal (*Prunella vulgaris*)   The herb is used both internally and externally. It has astringent properties and helps with sore mouths and throats. It can be mixed with honey and applied to wounds and ulcers after steeping for a few hours.

Strawberry (*Fragaria vesca*)   The leaves can be made into a pleasant sweet tea that has been used for dysentry. The fruit fruit rubbed over stained teeth will clean them. If sunburnt, rub on strawberries with a little honey. It makes a wonderfully soothing tonic.

Sunflower (*Helianthus annuus*)   Most parts of the plant are used. The seeds contain abundant oil which is used in cooking and cosmetics. The flowers contain abundant oil which is used in cooking and cosmetics. The flowers contain a yellow dye similar to that of the marigold. The seeds make a delicious nutritional snack and are used with great results in bronchial conditions.

Thyme, garden (*Thymus vulgaris*)   This herb is used in vinegar and salad dressings. The oil is distilled from the leaves and flowers and is used in aromatherapy to assist mucus in the body. It can be added to ointments for bruising and swelling.

Violet, sweet (*Viola odorata*)   The beautiful fragrance of the violet lends itself to the cosmetic industry. The whole plant is used medicinally. The fresh leaves can be taken internally as a tea, and may be used externally for poultices. The violet has been used with some success in cancer treatment of the tongue and throat.

Walnut (*Juglans nigra*)   The bark and leaves are used, particularly for skin disease and ulcers. By steeping walnut leaves for several hours, a tea for the skin can be made. The oil is obtained from the kernel and is used for cooking and skin preparations. It gives the hair a healthy sheen and is incorporated into soaps and shampoo on a commercial basis. It is said to benefit falling hair.

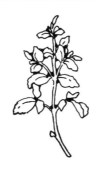

Watercress (*Nasturtium officinale*)   The leaves make a tasty addition to a salad. The juice expressed from the leaves assists in clearing up acne, possible due to its rich iron, sulphur and mineral content.

Witch hazel (*Hamamelis virginiana*)   This plant is mentioned frequently throughout this book for making cosmetics and toners. The dried bark and fresh and dried leaves are used, both yielding similar properties. Witch hazel is an astringent and acts on the fibres of the muscles. I find in my practice that it is excellent applied with cottonwool and left overnight for haemorrhoids. It reduces the swelling and soothes irritation. Dilute a little witch hazel with some glycerine and dab onto inflamed eyelids if they are red and itchy due to allergy or dust. The distillation of young leaves and twigs is utilised as a tea for internal conditions such as internal varicose veins. A poultice kept moist with witch hazel can be applied locally to swollen veins and brings great relief. It can be incorporated into creams and lotions for irritated, weepy skin conditions and keeps swellings and pain at bay. Mrs Grieve suggests a tea made from witch hazel after termination of a pregnancy to revitalise the system.

Yarrow (*Achillea millefolium*)   The Chinese used the stalks to predict the future. Yarrow has had many mystical connotations throughout history. The whole plant is used and is wonderful as a tonic to prevent falling hair. Internally it purifies the system and benefits the kidneys. It can be made into a tea and used as a facial astringent. It seems to assist in drawing blackheads and impurities from the skin.

Ylang-ylang (*Cananga odorata* or *Cananga odorata*)   The oil from this beautiful tree comes from the flowers. The quality depends on where it is cultivated. Those that come from the Philippines are said to be superior in quality. Ylang-ylang oil is soothing to the nervous system and when inhaled settles anger and frustration. Ylang-ylang added to your bath is very relaxing and luxurious. It is good for oily skin. Due to its lingering fragrance, it should be used in moderation. It is reputed to lower blood pressure and relieve anxiety. It has quite a strong sedating effect on the whole system. Add to herbal pillows or potpourris.

Definitions of Medical Terms

Absorptive	Capable of absorbing other substances
Acetylcholine	Fluid which transmits signals from one nerve ending to another
Alopecia	Loss of hair
Amenorrhoea	Absence of menstruation
Analgesic	A substance which relieves pain
Anodyne	A substance which relieves pain and/or soothes mentally
Anti-inflammatory	Reduces inflammation
Antiscorbutic	Effective in preventing or curing scurvy
Antiseptic	A substance which inhibits the growth of bacteria
Antispasmodic	Effective in preventing or curing spasms
Antivermitic	That which kills or expels worms from the body
Aperient	A mild laxative
Aromatic	Having a fragrant odour or spicy smell
Astringent	Causing contraction of muscular fibre or vessels
Bactericidal	A substance which inhibits or kills bacteria
Carminative	Expelling gas from the body and relieving flatulence
Cathartic	Stimulating the bowels; purgative
Demulcent	Soothing irritation and inflammation
Diuretic	Causing increased flow of urine
Emetic	Producing vomiting
Emollient	Softening and soothing
Expectorant	Relieving the bronchial tubes and lungs of mucus by inducing coughing or spitting
Febrifuge	Medicine to reduce fever
Fistula	An abnormal passage or duct formed by injury or disease
Hypotensive	Lowering blood pressure
Laxative	A mild stimulant for the bowel
Nervine	Relieving disorders of the nerves
Otitis	Inflammation of the ear

Parasiticide	Substance which kills parasites
Pectoral	Used internally to ease afflictions of the chest and lungs
Purgative	Purging or causing evacuation of the bowels
Quinsy	Inflammation of the throat
Rubefacient	A counter-irritant which produces redness or blisters on the skin
Sedative	Calming and sedating the nervous system
Stimulant	Increasing activity in the body or some part of it
Stomachic	Strengthens and tones the stomach
Stomatitis	Inflammation of the mucous membrane of the mouth
Sudorific	Promoting prolific perspiration
Tonic	Substance which restores health to the body or parts of it
Urticaria	Weals or itching of the skin (nettle rash)
Vulnerary	Used in healing wounds

Nutrient Chart

Nutrients	Bodily Action
Bioflavonoids	Help to increase strength of capillaries
Biotin	Necessary for carbohydrate, fat and protein metabolism. Aids in utilisation of other B group vitamins
Carbohydrate	Provides energy for body function and muscles. Assists in digestion and assimilation of foods
Choline	Important in nerve transmission, metabolism of fats. Helps regulate liver and gall
Fats	Provide energy, act as carriers for fat-soluble essential fatty acids needed for growth, health and smooth skin
Folic acid (folacin)	Important in red blood cell formation. Aids metabolism of protein necessary for growth and division of body cells
Inositol	Necessary for formation of lecithin connected with metabolism of fats including cholesterol. Vital for hair growth
Laetrile	Important in cancer prevention, although its use in treatment is controversial, and in some cases illegal
Niacin (nicotinic acid, niacinamide)	Maintains health of skin, tongue and digestive system. Essential for utilisation of carbohydrate fat and protein

Deficiency Symptoms	Source
Tendency to bleed and bruise easily	Citrus fruits, black currant, buckwheat
Dermatitis, greyish skin colour, depression, muscle pain, poor appetite	Egg yolk, liver, unpolished rice, brewer's yeast, whole grains, sardines, legumes
Loss of energy, fatigue, protein breakdown, imbalance of water, sodium potassium and chloride	Whole grains, sugar, honey, fruits and vegetables
Fatty liver, bleeding kidneys, high blood pressure	Soya beans, fish, legumes, lecithin, egg yolks
Eczema or skin disorders, retarded growth	Butter, vegetable oils, whole milk products, nuts
Poor growth, anaemia, vitamin B_{12} deficiency	Dark green leafy vegetables, organ meats, root vegetables, oysters, salmon, milk
Constipation, eczema, hair loss, cholesterol	Whole grains, citrus fruits, brewer's yeast molasses, meat, milk, nuts, vegetables
Diminished resistance to malignancies	Whole apricot kernels, apples, cherries, peaches, plums
Dermatitis, nervous disorders	Lean meats, poultry and fish, peanuts, rice bran, milk

Nutrients	Bodily Action
PABA (Para aminobenzoic acid)	Aids bacteria in production of folic acid. Acts as a co-enzyme in in the breakdown and utilisation of proteins. Aids in formation of red blood cells. Acts as a sunscreen.
Pangamic acid	Helps eliminate lyopscia. Assists in protein metabolism, stimulates nervous and glandular system
Pantothenic acid	Aids in formation of some fats, participates in the release of energy from carbohydrates, fats and protein. Improves body's resistance to stress
Protein	Essential for growth and development, formation of hormones, enzymes and antibodies; acid-alkali balance; heat and energy
Vitamin A	Necessary for growth and repair of body tissue, eyes and eyesight. Fights bacteria and infection, maintains healthy epithelial tissue, aids bone and teeth formation
Vitamin B (complex)	Necessary for carbohydrates, fat and protein metabolism. Helps functioning of the nervous system, muscle tone in gastro-intestinal tract
Vitamin B$_1$	Maintains health of skin, hair, eyes, mouth and liver. Necessary for carbohydrate metabolism. Maintains healthy nervous system. Stimulates growth and muscle tone

Deficiency Symptoms	Source
Fatigue, irritability, depression, nervousness, constipation, headache, digestive disorders, grey hair	Organ meats, wheat germ, yoghurt, molasses, green leafy vegetables
Diminished oxygenation of cells	Brewer's yeast, brown rice, sunflower, pumpkin and sesame seeds
Vomiting, restlessness, stomach stress, increased susceptibility to infection	Organ meats, brewer's yeast, egg yolk, legumes, whole grains, wheat germ, salmon
Fatigue, loss of appetite, diarrhoea and vomiting, stunted growth, oedema	Meat, fish, poultry, soya beans, eggs, milk, whole grains
Night blindness, rough, dry skin, fatigue, loss of smell and appetite	Fish liver oil, eggs, yellow fruits and vegetables
Dry, rough, cracked skin, acne, dull, dry or grey hair; fatigue, poor appetite, stomach disorders	Brewer's yeast
Gastro-intestinal problems, fatigue, loss of appetite, nerve disorders, heart disorders	Whole grains, molasses, brown rice, organ meats, egg yolks, nuts, brewer's yeast

Nutrients	Bodily Action
Vitamin B$_2$	Necessary for carbohydrate, fat and protein metabolism. Aids in formation of antibodies and red cells. Maintains respiration
Vitamin B$_6$ (pyridoxine)	Necessary for carbohydrate, fat and protein metabolism. Aids in formation of antibodies. Maintains balance of sodium and phosphorus
Vitamin B$_{12}$	Essential for normal formation of blood cells, for carbohydrate, fat and protein metabolism. Maintains nervous system
Vitamin B$_{13}$ (orotic acid)	Needed for metabolism of some B vitamins
Vitamin C	Maintains collagen, helps heal wounds, scar tissue and fractures. Gives strength to blood vessels. Provides resistance to stress
Vitamin D	Improves absorption, utilisation of calcium and phosphorus required for bone formation. Maintains stable nervous system and normal heart action
Vitamin E	Protects fat-soluble vitamins and red blood cells. Essential in cellular respiration. Inhibits coagulation of blood
Vitamin F	Important for respiration of vital organs. Helps maintain resilience and lubrication of cells. Helps regulate blood coagulation. Essential for normal glandular activity
Vitamin K	Necessary for blood coagulation

Deficiency Symptoms	Source
Eye problems, cracks and sores in mouth, dermatitis, retarded growth, digestive disturbances	Whole grains, brewer's yeast, legumes, nuts, egg yolks
Anaemia, mouth disorders, nervousness, muscular weakness, dermatitis, oedema and allergies	Meats, whole grains, organ meats, molasses, wheat germ, legumes, green leafy vegetables
Pernicious anaemia, brain damage, nervousness, neuritis	Organ meats, fish, pork, eggs, cheese, milk and milk products
Degenerative disorders	Root vegetables, whey
Bleeding gums, swollen or painful joints, slow healing of wounds and fractures, bruising, nosebleeds, impaired digestion	Citrus fruits, rose hips, alfalfa seeds, cantaloups, strawberries, broccoli, green peppers, tomoatoes
Vomiting, restlessness, stomach stress, increased susceptibility to infection	Salmon, sardines, herrings, vitamin D, fortified milk and milk products, egg yolk, organ meats
Rupture of red blood cells, muscular wasting, abnormal fat deposits in muscles	Cold-pressed oils, eggs, wheat germ, leafy vegetables, sesame seeds
Brittle, lustreless hair, brittle nails, dandruff, diarrhoea	Vegetable oil, butter, sunflower seeds
Increased tendency to haemorrhage and miscarriage	Green leafy vegetables, egg yolk, safflower oil

Mineral Chart

Mineral	Bodily Action
Calcium	Essential for development and maintenance of strong bones and teeth. Assists normal blood clotting, muscle action, nerve function and heart function
Chlorine	Regulates acid/base balance. Stimulates production of hydrochloric acid. Maintains joints and tendons
Chromium	Stimulates enzymes in metabolism of energy and synthesis of fatty acids
Cobalt	Functions as part of vitamin B_{12}. Maintains red blood cells. Activates a number of enzymes in the body
Copper	Aids in formation of red blood cells. Forms part of many enzymes. Works with vitamin C to form elastin
Fluorine	May reduce tooth decay by discouraging the growth of acid-forming bacteria
Iodine	Essential part of the hormone thyroxine. Necessary for prevention of goitre. Regulates energy and metabolism. Promotes growth
Iron	Necessary for haemoglobin and myoglobin formation. Helps protein metabolism. Promotes growth
Magnesium	Acts as a catalyst in the utilisation of carbohydrates, fats, protein, calcium, phosphorus and potassium

Deficiency Symptoms	Source
Softening of bones, back and leg pains, brittle bones	Milk and milk products, green leafy vegetables, shellfish, molasses
Loss of hair and teeth, poor muscular contractibility	Seafood, meat, olives, rye flour
Depressed growth rate, glucose intolerance in diabetics, atherosclerosis	Corn oil, whole grain cereals, brewer's yeast
Pernicious anaemia, slow rate of growth	Oysters, clams, poultry, green vegetables, milk, fruits
General weakness, impaired respiration, skin sores	Organ meats, seafood, nuts, legumes, raisins
Tooth decay	Tea, seafood, fluoridated water
Weakness, paleness of skin, constipation, anaemia	Pineapple, green leafy vegetables, egg yolks
Weakness, paleness of skin, constipation anaemia	Meat, eggs, fish, poultry, green leafy vegetables, dried fruits
Nervousness, muscular excitability, tremors	Seafood, whole grains, dark green vegetables, nuts

Mineral	Bodily Action
Manganese	Activates enzymes. Necessary for normal skeletal development. Maintains sex hormone production
Molybdenum	Acts in oxidation of fats and aldehydes. Aids in mobilisation of iron from liver reserves
Phosphorus	Works with calcium to build bones and teeth. Utilises carbohydrates, fats and proteins
Potassium	Works to control activity of heart muscles, nervous system and kidneys
Selenium	Works with vitamin E. Preserves tissue elasticity
Sodium	Maintains normal fluid levels in cells. Maintains health of the nervous, muscular, blood and lymph systems
Sulphur	Necessary for collagen synthesis and formation of body tissue. Part of vitamin B and amino acid role
Zinc	Is a component of insulin and male reproductive fluid. Aids in healing process

Deficiency Symptoms	Source
Paralysis, convulsions, dizziness, ataxia, blindness and deafness in infants	Whole grains, green leafy vegetables, legumes, nuts, pineapple, egg yolks
Premature aging	Legumes, whole grain cereals, milk and liver
Loss of weight and appetite, irregular breathing, pyorrhoea	Fish, meats, poultry, eggs, milk and milk products, nuts, whole grain cereals
Poor reflexes, respiratory failure, cardiac arrest	Lean meats, whole grains, vegetables, dried fruits, legumes, sunflower seeds
Premature aging	Tuna, herring, brewer's yeast, wheat germ, bran, broccoli, whole grains
Muscle weakness and shrinkage, nausea and general loss of appetite, wind and gas in bowel and stomach	Seafood, table salt, celery, milk products
Infections, poor memory	Fish, eggs, meat, cabbage, brussels sprouts
Retarded growth, hair and nail weakness, delayed sexual maturity	Pumpkin seeds, sunflower seeds, mushrooms, brewer's yeast, soya beans

Weights and Measures

Abbreviations

tsp	=	teaspoon
tbsp	=	tablespoon
ml	=	millilitre
fl oz	=	fluid ounce
g	=	gram or grams
oz	=	ounce
lb	=	pound

Apothecaries Weight

20 grains	=	1 scruple		
3 scruples	=	1 dram	=	60 grains
8 drams	=	1 ounce	=	480 grains
12 ounces	=	1 pound	=	5760 grains

Avoirdupois Weight

27+ grains	=	1 dram		
16 drams	=	1 ounce	=	473+ grains
16 ounces	=	1 pound	=	7000 grains

Useful Equivalents

15 grains	=	¼ teaspoon
20 grains	=	⅓ teaspoon
60 grains	=	1 teaspoon
1 teaspoon	=	⅓ tablespoon or 60 grains or 5 grams or 3 scruples
1 tablespoon	=	3 teaspoons or 15 grams or ½ ounce
1 ml	=	12 drops
5 ml	=	60 drops or 1 teaspoon or 1 dram
15 ml	=	3 teaspoons or 1 tablespoon
28 ml	=	6 teaspoons or 2 tablespoons or 1 fluid ounce
224 ml	=	16 tablespoons or 8 fluid ounces
452 ml	=	16 fluid ounces
1134 ml	=	1.134 litres (40 fluid ounces)
.08 g	=	1 grain = 1 drop
1 g	=	12 grains = 12 drops
453.6 g	=	1 lb
1000 g	=	2.2 lb = 1 kg

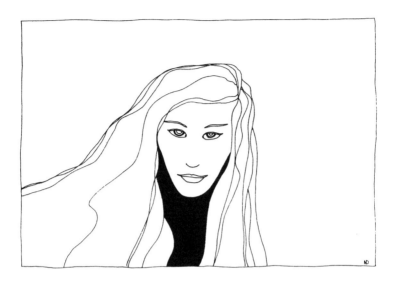

BIBLIOGRAPHY

Bayne, Murdo MacDonald, *Heal Yourself*, L. N. Fowler & Co., Essex 1947

Buchman, Dian Dincin, *Feed Your Face*, Duckworth, London 1973

Douglas, James Shotto, *Making Your Own Cosmetics*, Pelham Books, London 1979

Francke, Elizabeth, *Cosmetic and Fragrance Book*, Doubleday, Sydney 1982

Grieve, M., *A Modern Herbal*, Dover, New York 1971

Guyton, Anita, *The Book of Natural Beauty*, Stanley Paul & Co., London 1981

Hall, Dorothy, *The Book of Herbs*, Angus and Robertson, Sydney 1983

Hopkins, Albert A., *The Standard American Encyclopaedia of Formulas*, Grosset and Dunlap, New York 1953

Lautie, Raymond, and Passeberg, André, *Aromatherapy*, Thorsons, Northamptonshire 1979

Lusher, Max, *Colour Test*, Jonathan Cape, London 1969

Meredith, Bronwen, *Vogue Body and Beauty Book*, A & W Publishers, New York 1981

Meyer, Joseph, *The Herbalist*, Meyerbooks, Illinois 1976

Rose, Jeanne, *Herbs and Things*, Grosset and Dunlap, New York 1974

Tisserand, Maggie, *Aromatherapy for Women*, Thorsons Publishers, Northamptonshire 1985

Tisserand, Robert, *The Art of Aromatherapy*, C. W. Daniel, London 1977

*Illustrations pages 92, 93 and 162
courtesy of Nevill Drury*